Nutrition in Catering

Nutrition in Catering

The impact of nutrition and health concepts on catering practice

Edited by Richard Cottrell

Proceedings of the Seventh
British Nutrition Foundation Annual Conference

The Parthenon Publishing Group
International Publishers in Science & Technology

Casterton Hall, Carnforth,
Lancs, LA6 2LA, U.K.

120 Mill Road, Park Ridge,
New Jersey, U.S.A.

Published in the UK and Europe by
The Parthenon Publishing Group Limited,
Casterton Hall, Carnforth,
Lancs. LA6 2LA, England.

Published in the USA by
The Parthenon Publishing Group Inc.,
120 Mill Road,
Park Ridge,
New Jersey 07656

ISBN 1 85070 123 7

First published 1987

Typeset by Lonsdale Typesetting Services,
Burton-in-Lonsdale, Carnforth, Lancashire

Printed in Great Britain by
Antony Rowe Ltd., Chippenham

Contents

Acknowledgements

The Foundation wishes to express its appreciation of the help given during the planning of the Huddersfield Conference by Professor George Glew and the staff of the Department of Catering Studies, Huddersfield Polytechnic, particularly John Dawson.

We are also grateful to all those who agreed to speak at the conference and to provide papers for publication, to Judith Dutton for the preparation of the manuscript and to the Parthenon Publishing Group for their co-operation in the publishing of this book.

List of contributors

T. A. Ball
Senior Catering Adviser,
Department of Education and Science,
Elizabeth House,
39 York Road,
London SE1 7PH

J. Dockerty
Procter Department of Food Science,
The University of Leeds,
Woodhouse Lane,
Leeds,
West Yorkshire LS2 9JT

G. Glew
Professor, Hotel and Catering Research Centre,
Catering Studies Department,
Huddersfield Polytechnic,
Huddersfield,
West Yorkshire HD1 3DH

G. Heald
Joint Managing Director,
Social Surveys (Gallup Poll) Limited,
202 Finchley Road,
London NW3 6BL

A. R. Horton
Chief Officer on Catering and Dietetics,
Department of Health and Social Security,
Hannibal House,
Elephant and Castle,
London SE1 6TE

C. Hunt
Hotel and Catering Research Centre,
Catering Studies Department,
Huddersfield Polytechnic,
Huddersfield,
West Yorkshire HD1 3DH

J. Lawson
Hotel and Catering Research Centre,
Catering Studies Department,
Huddersfield Polytechnic,
Huddersfield,
West Yorkshire HD1 3DH

J. Pascoe
Procter Department of Food Science,
The University of Leeds,
Woodhouse Lane,
Leeds, West Yorkshire LS2 9JT

J. Ryley
Procter Department of Food Science,
The University of Leeds,
Woodhouse Lane,
Leeds, West Yorkshire LS2 9JT

R. Skinner,
Senior Medical Officer,
Head of Nutrition Unit,
Department of Health and Social Security,
Alexander Fleming House,
Elephant and Castle,
London SE1 6BY

E. M. Widdowson
Department of Medicine,
Addenbrooke's Hospital,
Hills Road,
Cambridge CB2 2QQ

Foreword

Catering — the changing scene

In recent years the provision of food by caterers has come under the scrutiny of those who are interested to change eating patterns within the UK. It is not that many people consume an important part of their weekly food from a particular catering establishment; few do. On the contrary, it is because of a constantly changing clientele that the hotelier, restaurateur or catering manager can exert such an influence on popular eating habits. It is the prospect of using the caterers as a tool to influence large numbers of individuals that excites the attention of those whose aim is to improve the health of the people by changing their diet. Thus, hospital kitchens (both for patients and staff), schools, colleges, works and office canteens, restaurants and hotels, are being urged to provide food which conforms to the current nutritional thinking as to what is healthy. It is left to the executive to ensure customer satisfaction.

Against this background, the British Nutrition Foundation devoted its 1985 Annual Conference to the subject 'Nutrition in Catering — the Impact of Nutrition and Health Concepts on Catering Practice' and chose as a venue one of the foremost research schools in catering technology — Huddersfield Polytechnic. The papers presented at the conference discuss the various facets of the catering industry and the complex interactions between what is technically or organisationally feasible on the one hand, and what the consumer appears to be prepared to accept on the other.

In order to provide the reader of this volume with as comprehensive a reference work as possible, the opening chapter reproduces a summary paper, produced by the Foundation earlier in 1985, which discusses the available evidence on the effects of catering methods on the nutritional quality of the food ultimately provided to the consumer.

R. C. Cottrell

The British Nutrition Foundation
15 Belgrave Square
London SW1X 8PS

July 1986

1
Nutrition in catering

INTRODUCTION

This chapter is intended to provide a summary of current information on the effects of catering methods on the nutrient content of food as consumed. It is confined to methods and circumstances of food provision which differ from domestic techniques, and includes only foods consumed at or near the point of sale or delivery. Thus, traditional catering outlets (hospitals, prisons, the armed forces, residential homes, schools, large restaurants and hotels, canteens, etc.), fast-food and take-away establishments, airlines and 'Meals on Wheels' are included; small restaurants, which may use essentially domestic methods and ingredients, are not. Consideration of microbiological aspects of food preparation methods is largely excluded from this chapter.

Current public interest in health and nutrition has introduced new elements into customer demands of commercial catering establishments and scrutiny of the performance of the non-profit-making sector. The catering manager is thus faced with a new and additional responsibility to provide clients with the option of dishes of different composition from those traditionally served. Increasingly, 'low-calorie', fat-reduced and high fibre dishes are an expected feature of menus and the customary level of the use of salt as a seasoning is being loudly criticised in some quarters. Whether or not these perceptions of 'healthy eating' prove to be soundly based, it is unlikely that they can be wholly ignored by the catering manager in the near future.

The Report of the Committee on Medical Aspects of Food Policy on *Diet in Relation to Cardiovascular Disease* (1984) has recommended a reduction in fat and saturated fat consumption to 35% and 15% of food energy respectively by individuals whose intake is in excess of these levels. The view taken in the report was that there was sufficient consistency in the evidence available 'to make it more likely than not that the incidence of coronary heart disease will be reduced' by decreasing the intake of saturated fatty acids and total fat. This report emphasises the necessity for caterers to provide information on the composition of foods so that individuals who may wish to adjust their intake of particular dietary components are able to do so (DHSS, 1984).

The provision of large numbers of meals or snacks essentially simultaneously, or at any rate with a minimum of delay, makes special demands upon an establishment. Techniques of preparation, storage and cooking have to be modified from those of an ordinary domestic situation, and the drive to reduce labour costs has led to the development of a range of pre-packaged and prepared foods designed for this market.

The nutrient content of foodstuffs provided by a caterer may differ from a well prepared home-cooked meal both because the preparation, storage and cooking methods differ and also because of the choice and composition of available ingredients and supplies. Either facet may lead to important differences in nutrient content but neither, in principle, need lead to serious changes. Methods are available which will allow nutritionally valuable meals to be provided and any public demand for a particular balance of nutrient content can be met. Any meal provided should contain the nutrients to be expected from its constituent foodstuffs.

The ability to distribute meals of adequate and appropriate nutrient composition is of particular importance where the food provided by the caterer represents a significant proportion of the daily consumption of an individual. For example, in hospitals the patients will receive essentially all their food from the hospital caterers and careful attention to detail is clearly required to ensure adequate levels of nutrient provision and avoidance of excesses (Lawson, Hunt and Glew, 1983). Within the National Health Service in 1982–3, 312 million meals were produced for patients, and a count of school meals in England showed that they were provided for 3.48 million children (51.4% of those present at school) on a single day in the autumn of 1983.

This chapter is presented in three sections:

(1) General aspects of effects of large-scale cooking on nutrients in food.
(2) Catering methods: the sensitive areas.
(3) Recommendations for caterers.

GENERAL ASPECTS OF EFFECTS OF LARGE-SCALE COOKING ON NUTRIENTS IN FOOD

Fats

The choice of cooking method may have a significant effect on the fat content of the food provided by a caterer. Grilling on a rack, for example, will lead to a reduction of the fat content of meat and meat products. Deep frying, on the other hand, may increase fat content substantially. When saturated fats (for example, lard) are used, the product may absorb saturated fat. Unsaturated oils (for example, corn oil) may be preferable, particularly for individuals who wish to lower their dietary intake of saturated fat.

Deterioration of fats may occur as a result of oxidation during heating in air but is unlikely to be of significance nutritionally. The minor resulting change in energy value is unlikely to be important in most circumstances. Losses of essential fatty acids (which may form part of the fat structures) are unlikely to be important except for individuals on an exceptionally low fat diet. Unsaturated fatty acids are more readily oxidised than saturated ones and consequently fats and oils rich in unsaturated fatty acids are more prone to oxidative change than their saturated counterparts, unless protected by natural or synthetic antioxidants.

Two disadvantages of fat oxidation, however, cannot be wholly ignored. Firstly, the oxidation process can exacerbate damage to fat-soluble vitamins, particularly vitamin A (see below). Secondly, the products of oxidation may be undesirable in themselves, although the evidence for this seems inconclusive.

The consequences of fat oxidation in terms of off-flavours in the food are likely to limit the acceptable level of accumulation of oxidation products in cooking fats and oils in most catering practice. Fat oxidation, which may be detected as undesirable off-flavours, can also occur during chilled and frozen storage of fatty foods and limits shelf life.

Protein

The amino-acid components of protein which are nutritionally essential include the sulphur-containing amino-acids. These are oxidised on heating or prolonged exposure to air. Losses have been shown to occur even at −18 °C under nitrogen, over a prolonged period. Losses of another essential amino-acid, lysine, can also occur as a result of heat-dependent browning reactions in the presence of, for example, sugars. Furthermore, excessive heating will cause losses by cross-linking reactions, for example, in roasting or baking. Alkaline cooking conditions will accelerate oxidation and cross-linking of a number of amino-acids, causing them to become nutritionally unavailable. Small amounts of protein may also be lost in the drip from meat and fish on thawing. These losses are unlikely, however, to be significant for most people.

Carbohydrates

The losses of digestible carbohydrates (starches and sugars) which may occur during heating of food are not usually considered important in themselves in relation to nutrition. Undesirable flavours may result from overheating but, since carbohydrates constitute but one of many sources of energy in the diet, the minor losses deriving from, for example, leaching into the cooking water are not serious. Starch is generally more readily digested following cooking.

Dietary fibre

An adequate choice of menu items which contain the various forms of dietary fibre (for example, bread, cereals, potatoes, vegetables, fruit) will ensure that consumers are able to select foods which provide this component in their diet.

During cooking these foods may undergo changes in texture and hence in eating quality. These changes may improve general palatability without significant loss of physiological value of the dietary fibre they contain. Excessive cooking, however, may cause losses of soluble nutrients which are partly dependent upon the changes in dietary fibre structures which enclose other cellular constituents.

Vitamins

Vitamin loss

Water-soluble vitamins (the B group and C) may be lost during cooking, particularly by leaching into water used in the preparation of vegetables. The level of certain vitamins, for example vitamin C, may be reduced additionally as a result of destruction by oxidation or enzyme action. Consequently, re-use of cooking liquor will be only partially effective in returning some stable, water-soluble, vitamins into the meal; for example, thiamin (vitamin B_1) and vitamin B_6 (pyridoxine and derivatives). Avoidance of excessive cooking or warmholding time will minimise losses by oxidation, and rapid blanching of vegetables will minimise enzyme-dependent breakdown of vitamins.

Riboflavin (vitamin B_2) is light-sensitive and destroyed by heat. In alkaline conditions, the breakdown products of riboflavin may, in turn, destroy vitamin C. Small doses of riboflavin in milk (for example, 5%) may, by this mechanism, lead to substantial losses of vitamin C (as much as 50%) (Bender, 1978). Fat-soluble vitamins (A, D, E, K) may be damaged by the processes (heat, air) which accelerate the rate of fat oxidation in foods. Vitamin A is particularly susceptible, and so is its precursor carotene (which is responsible for the orange colour in many vegetables). Since the oxidation process is autocatalytic — that is, once started it accelerates — care should be taken to avoid fat oxidation where possible. Prolonged storage at low temperatures may be equivalent in this respect to short periods at high temperatures.

In contrast, cooking may in some circumstances increase the concentration of the nutritionally available form of a vitamin in a food. An example is found in the improvement of niacin availability on baking cereal products, particularly in alkaline conditions (for example, in making tortilla from maize).

Use of ascorbate as index of loss of nutrients

Vitamin C (ascorbic acid, ascorbate) is frequently measured in foods in order to provide information on process-dependent losses of nutrients. This vitamin is particularly sensitive to oxidation, leaching and enzyme catalysed losses, and consequently has a certain value as an indicator for process control. It is not, however, typical of other nutrients and should not be taken as a measure of loss of other components. While adequate retention of vitamin C may indicate correctly that the food has not be adversely affected by the treatment to which it has been subjected, the converse is not necessarily true. Losses of vitamin C can occur without concomitant losses of other components.

Only in foodstuffs which are significant contributors to vitamin C intake should loss of vitamin C itself be considered as a serious issue. The contribution of potatoes (19% of total) and vegetables

Table 1.1 Nutrient losses during preparation, cooking and service of animal and vegetable products

Food affected	*Process involved*	*Loss caused by*	*Examples of nutrients lost*
Animal products			
Chopped or ground meats, fish	Freeze-thaw	Thaw drip	Protein, B vitamins, particularly niacin (nicotinic acid)
Meat joints	Microwave cooking, grilling, roasting	Cooking drip	Fat, fat-soluble vitamins
All	Braising or stewing	Leaching	Water-soluble vitamins
All	Heat (either prolonged or to a high temperature) as in roasting, baking, warmholding	Oxidation or breakdown of nutrients	Thiamin, essential amino-acids and fatty acids
Plant products			
Fruit, vegetables	Bruising, prolonged storage	Spoilage in unprocessed state	Vitamin C
Fruit, vegetables	Trimming, cutting, chopping of raw materials	Disruption of cellular architecture	Vitamin C
All	Cooking, washing, soaking in water	Leaching of water-soluble components	Vitamin C, thiamin, folate, pyridoxine
All	Heat (either prolonged or to a high temperature) as in roasting, baking, warmholding	Oxidation or breakdown of nutrients	Vitamin C, riboflavin, essential fatty acids and amino-acids
All	Discarded cooking water	Leaching	Vitamin C, thiamin, riboflavin, zinc
Cereals, green vegetables	Alkali in soaking or cooking	Oxidation enhanced	Thiamin, riboflavin, vitamin C
Fruit and vegetables	Prolonged refrigeration or cooked material	Oxidation	Vitamin C

in general (47%) to total household consumption of vitamin C (MAFF, 1985) is considerable, however. It may legitimately be claimed, therefore, that losses of vitamin C from vegetables during catering-specific processes are likely to be nutritionally significant, particularly to 'captive' consumer groups. Indeed, there has been some evidence of this in long-stay hospital patients (Lawson, Hunt, and Glew, 1983).

Minerals

Losses of minerals will occur by leaching into cooking water (for example, potassium, iron), while the use of salt in cooking will lead to an increase in sodium content. It is generally unlikely that such effects will be nutritionally important but they may have significance in particular groups. For example, loss of iron from vegetables may have little effect on people whose main intake comes from meat, but may be important to the vegetarian. Conversely, the rise in sodium content may be important to those individuals whose intake is already excessive. Minerals are assumed to be stable to cooking.

Energy

Changes in the energy content of food may occur during cooking when changes in physical composition occur. Examples are fat losses during grilling, which will lower energy content, and fat absorption during frying, which will raise it.

The main causes of nutrient loss are summarised in Table 1.1.

CATERING METHODS: THE SENSITIVE AREAS

Conventional catering

In the traditional systems, still operated by a large number of enterprises, large-scale preparation and cooking of foodstuffs is followed by a period of holding at warm temperature prior to service. In order to ensure microbiological safety, the warmholding must (by law) be conducted so that the food is maintained at 62.7 °C or above (HMSO, 1970). If re-heating before service is to be avoided, then the acceptability of hot food to the consumer also requires an adequate temperature for this process. However, it has been frequently observed in surveys that food produced in this way is not always as hot as it might be (Lawson, 1982).

Since losses of certain nutrients during cooking and warmholding may be considerable, particular attention needs to be given to the need to minimise both cooking and warmholding time and temperature. In both cases, these nutritional considerations may conflict with those involved in the choice of conditions which may produce the most acceptable eating quality of the product and, more importantly, ensure microbiological safety. A compromise must therefore be reached. While neither taste nor nutritional value of foodstuffs is improved by excessive cooking time or temperature, adequate cooking is essential for many foodstuffs. A certain amount of browning during cooking is generally considered desirable for many dishes, despite the consequent loss of nutritional value (Bender, 1978).

Cook-freeze

One development in catering methods which has practical advantages to the caterer, and may also lead to a nutritionally superior product, involves the rapid freezing of food after cooking. Storage and, if required, distribution may then be undertaken in the frozen state (−18 °C), followed by re-heating at the point of service. This technique allows food manufacturers and caterers to produce essentially complete menus for distribution frozen and, if properly operated, will lead to a supply of food to the consumer which has not been subject to the prolonged exposure to raised temperatures which might otherwise be required. An example of the superior

Table 1.2 Vitamin C content of vegetables in two catering systems

Food (system)	*Mean value* (mg/100 g)	*Range of value* (mg/100 g)	*Number of observations*
Peas			
(conventional)	1.8	0.3– 4.0	7
(cook-freeze)	12.5[a]	8.4–19.7	10
New potatoes			
(conventional)	8.6	5.5–11.3	6
(cook-freeze)	20.3[a]	10.3–32.2	10
Cabbage			
(conventional)	5.0	1.2– 7.7	10
(cook-freeze)	12.8[a]	3.9–28.2	14

[a] Significantly different from conventional system, $p < 0.01$.
(From Glew, Hill and Millross, 1971)

retention of one nutrient, ascorbic acid (vitamin C), which can be achieved in a cook-freeze operation when compared with conventional methods, is given in Table 1.2. The improvement is only achieved when the exposure to water and heat is minimised by strict adherence to good processing procedures. (DHSS guidelines on cook-freeze methods are expected to be published shortly).

Cook-chill

Another alternative to conventional catering methods is provided by the 'cook-chill' approach. This method differs from 'cook-freeze' in two important respects. Firstly, the food is stored at +2 °C following cooking and subsequent rapid chilling before re-heating for service to the consumer. In consequence, the energy costs are lower than for cook-freeze. It has also been claimed that less recipe adaptation is required in the cook-chill method. Secondly, the maximum storage time at +2 °C will clearly be shorter than at −18 °C for reasons of bacteriological safety. The DHSS

Table 1.3 Percentage vitamin C retention in cooked/frozen vegetables thawed to +5 °C in a rapid thaw cabinet and then stored at +5 °C for up to 48 hours

Vegetable	*Thawing time* (h)	*% retention after 24 h at 5 °C*	*% retention after 48 h at 5 °C*
Peas	3	98	72
Beans	3	—	85
Cauliflower	3¾	69	65
Sprouts	3¾	—	81
Cabbage	4	89	87
Potatoes	4	78	54

(From Hunt, 1984)

guidelines on precooked chilled foodstuffs (1980) specify a maximum storage time of 5 days at +2 °C (0 to +3 °C) (this includes the day of cooking and the day of serving). Significant nutrient losses may occur during storage at +2 °C, however (see Table 1.3), which may account in part for the 30–90% loss of vitamin C seen in the final meal (Bognar, 1980). These losses are largely due to exposure to oxygen in the air during refrigerated storage and could be minimised in sensitive products by storage in the absence of oxygen. Furthermore, unsaturated fat can be oxidised in food, causing a flavour change in products high in unsaturated fat. These changes have been reviewed by Hunt (1984) and Glew (1980), who both concluded that in properly operated systems the cook-freeze method was likely to provide meals of higher nutrient content than those normally produced by either conventional or cook-chill methods.

Cook-freeze methods have the additional advantage of a greater resilience to malpractice, particularly as regards temperature control, although it should be emphasised that poor attention to storage conditions may have serious consequences in terms of microbiological safety. A combination of the two systems may provide the best solution to many catering problems.

Cook-freeze-thaw

A modification of cook-freeze involves rapid thawing of frozen foodstuffs to +2 °C. Thereafter the method is identical both in advantages and limitations to the cook-chill method.

Convenience methods

All branches and techniques of catering practice are increasingly dependent upon convenience products for their operation because of the cost implications of labour in the kitchen. A variety of pre-prepared materials is available, ranging from single commodities to complete meals. One impact of these technological developments is to shift the burden of responsibility for the nutritional content of the foods away from the caterer towards the manufacturer. If pre-packaged and cooked products are to be extensively used in the provision of food to those who will rely heavily on these meals for their nutrition, the producer of the packs must accept a responsibility to ensure a nutritionally desirable balance in the meals.

For some children, school meals make a significant contribution to their nutritional requirements. It is therefore particularly useful to consider the comparison of traditional catering and convenience methods in school meal preparation provided by Ryley (1984). This comparison is, however, somewhat difficult to make since certain convenience items, for example, dried skimmed milk, are now so established as to be considered traditional. This study highlighted the importance of accurate information on ingredients in order that the caterer can plan nutritionally desirable meals. Differences in the provision of other nutrients for a given level of energy in the meals were also apparent; the convenience meals, for example, generally supplying less iron, riboflavin (vitamin B_2) and calcium for a given energy content and more sodium, ascorbic acid (vitamin C) and water. Some of these differences were attributed to the use of particular commodities in traditional methods of preparation. The poor vitamin C content of traditionally prepared meals was thought to be caused by the methods used, which involved fine chopping of cabbage, prolonged mashing of potatoes and warmholding.

Fast food

This description refers more to a marketing method than to a system of catering, but in general fits into the convenience method bracket. Fast food outlets rely upon a choice of convenience foodstuffs which are in a form ready for rapid regeneration into an attractive product. At present, in the UK, consumption of such foods does not represent a substantial proportion of the average nutritional intake of most people. It seems likely, however, that some consumers may rely heavily upon such meals and that future

Table 1.4 Comparison of some typical fast food meals

Meal	*Portion (weight)* (g)	*Protein* (g)	*Carbo-hydrate* (g)	*Fat* (g)	*Energy*[c] (MJ)	*Energy from fat* (%)
Hamburger[a] with French fries	182	15.5	58.8	25.8	2.2	44.2
Cheeseburger[a] with French fries	196	17.5	59.6	29.0	2.4	46.8
Hamburger[a] with French fries, apple pie	272	18.3	93.9	40.0	3.3	45.0
Cheeseburger[a] with French fries, apple pie	286	20.3	94.7	44.1	3.5	46.7
Haddock[b] fried in batter with chips	299	24.7	62.6	38.8	2.9	50.2
Beef Chow Mein[b] with noodles	557	37.3	61.3	29.5	2.7	40.3
Pizza[b] (cheese and tomato)	351	49.8	120.0	33.4	4.0	30.8

[a] Data on each meal are means of six independent outlets
[b] Data on each meal are means of six outlets in the Leeds area. (From Pascoe, Docherty, and Ryley, personal communication)
[c] 1 MJ = 239 kcal

trends will be towards increased consumption of these forms of foodstuffs.

The restricted range of menu items, and the choice of foodstuffs which are amenable to the cooking methods used, may mean that meals from such outlets are somewhat high in fat. Table 1.4 shows some average analytical results obtained on typical fast food meals (Pascoe, Docherty and Ryley, personal communication). The percentage energy from fat is higher than for some other types of meal. Thus, people who frequently eat meals of this kind may need to balance their diet by eating less fatty foods at other meals. Fat has more than twice the energy value of protein and carbohydrate and regular consumption of high fat foods is likely to lead to weight gain. Certain aspects of the techniques used, however, are amenable to changes that would reduce the amount of energy provided by these meals. The fat content of chips, for example, can be reduced by making chunky rather than thin chips, provided small loads are fried so that the oil temperature recovers rapidly after addition of the chips. An increase in the dietary fibre content of the diet would be beneficial to some people. Meals of the type included in Table 1.4 are somewhat low in dietary fibre, but could be improved in this regard by the use of wholemeal buns or the inclusion of salads containing components such as peas, beans, nuts, carrots and cabbage.

The quality of oil or fat used for frying is a matter of concern. It is an expensive commodity whose life must be as long as possible for economy. However, oils which have been heated for too long a period not only impart undesirable colour and flavour to foods, they also contain breakdown products which may be detrimental. Therefore, oils must not be used when they have deteriorated excessively. Chemical methods of testing the extent of oil breakdown exist and are of some help in making a decision to replace the oil in a fryer. In the absence of such help, oil should not be allowed to foam or impart dark colours and off-flavours to the food. The life of frying oil can be extended by using small fryers with continuous throughput so that oil is removed rapidly from the fryers by the food and thus the oil is not stored hot but unused for long periods. Regular filtering to remove food particles is essential.

RECOMMENDATIONS FOR CATERERS

Provision of uncooked fruit and vegetables

Provision of a selection of uncooked fruit and vegetables is an increasing and welcome feature of catering practice. Spoilage of chopped or cut plant products is a familiar feature of kitchen life. What may be less commonly appreciated is the loss of nutrients which can occur on storage which does not lead to noticeable spoilage or change in taste both in whole fruits and vegetables and in the cut state.

Losses of vitamin C may occur due to air oxidation and other processes. These may be minimised by limiting storage time, use of chilled storage, and avoiding excessive handling which may lead to bruising. If the materials are to be served in a cut form (chopped, sliced, etc.), this should be carried out as close to the time of serving as possible, since enzyme catalysed destruction of vitamin C, for example, will be accelerated by the disruption of cellular architecture involved in this process. Refrigeration is recommended for maintaining both nutritional quality and texture of cut fruit and vegetables. Coarse chopping is less damaging than fine, but is limited by consumer acceptability. Prolonged soaking in water will leach out water-soluble vitamins and should be avoided.

Provision of cooked food

Conventional methods

The characteristic of conventional catering methods which has most nutritional implication is excessively long periods of heating to which food may be exposed. Losses of a number of nutrients occur in direct relation to the time of heating and temperature used. Thus, for example, boiling a large quantity of vegetables in an inadequately heated vessel may require a very long time. Vegetables near the heat source may be exposed to temperatures high enough to reduce the level of certain vitamins. Equally, an excessively long period in a bain marie or hot cupboard may lead to reduction in some vitamins, oxidation of protein components and peroxidation of fats. These processes can have unpleasant effects on the eating quality of food in addition to reducing its nutrional value.

Modern techniques

Attempts to compare the merits of conventional, cook-freeze and cook-chill techniques have generally tended to support the proposition that the more modern techniques offer significant nutritional improvements over conventional methods. Of the new techniques, cook-freeze has many practical and nutritional advantages, particularly when carried out to conform to the best practice. Cook-chill catering also has advantages, but attention should be given to oxidation in the food and hence possible loss of nutrients; as the system is currently used. There is little disagreement among experimenters that excessive warmholding should be avoided and that catering practice should be designed to minimise this undesirable feature of conventional techniques (Lawson, Hunt and Glew, 1983).

Fast foods

Fast foods have received particular attention, not because of loss of nutrients, for which this method of preparation has distinct advantages, but because of concern that they may lack certain nutrients and contain too much of others. Typical fast food outlets provide a range of foods which can be purchased in any desired combination. It is quite possible, therefore, to select an inappropriate balance of items from a nutritional point of view. This is, however, not a new phenomenon and is equally true for captive consumers. A traditional school meal, for example, may have been nutritionally admirable (when devised) but the child may have selected only part of it to eat. Nonetheless, it has been suggested that some fast food products may be too rich in fat and salt (sodium) and that excessive consumption of these products may consequently have an effect on the overall diet of certain individuals (Ryley, 1981). These problems may be of particular significance to the school child, but are confined to a limited number of nutrients (Ryley, 1983, 1984). Fast food caterers should seek to provide a balance of nutrients among their products.

Provided a suitable variety of foods is offered and information and guidance are available (for example, in leaflet form), consumers will be able to make their individual choice of an appropriate meal or snack which fits into their overall dietary habits.

Microwave

Microwave cooking has been reviewed by Cross and Fung (1982), who concluded that this method of cooking is comparable to traditional techniques from the nutritional point of view. In certain catering operations, however, it is possible that the use of microwave cooking could avoid the necessity of warmholding. Under these circumstances, this form of cooking may confer nutritional advantages.

Provision of cold cooked foods

Although the problems of warmholding or reheating of cooked food are avoided if the food is subsequently served cold, it should not be assumed that all losses of nutrients are halted once cooked food is cooled to storage temperature. Storage at +2 °C can lead to losses in certain foods, particularly if prolonged (as already mentioned in relation to cook-chill methods). Storage at −18 °C may offer considerable advantages but does not avoid all losses of nutrients. Exposure of cooked foods to sunlight or temperatures above +2 °C, as in an unrefrigerated display, may lead to changes in nutritive value. These changes are likely, however, to be overshadowed by microbiological spoilage.

CONCLUSION

Catering methods and the choice of commodities used in preparation can have significant effects on the nutrient content and balance of the foodstuffs provided. Adequate attention to technique can avoid unnecessary loss of nutrient quality during preparation, storage, cooking and distribution to the recipient. Careful choice of ingredients, and formulation, could dispel current anxieties of less than optimal nutritional balance in some types of meals. The increased reliance of caterers on pre-prepared convenience forms of catering supplies brings with it an obligation upon the manufacturer to seek sound professional advice on the composition of the foodstuffs produced and the consequences of the methods of preparation used.

The COMA Report (DHSS, 1984) suggests that information on the composition of foodstuffs provided by the caterer should be made available to the consumer so that an individual choice of the dietary intake of various nutrients can be made. This is particularly important in relation to fat content, and menu options low in fat (and labelled as such) should be made available, since this will allow individuals who wish to follow a lower fat diet to do so.

Acknowledgement

This chapter was published in February 1985 as the *British Nutrition Foundation Briefing Paper No. 4*, and is reproduced with permission.

References

Bender, A. E. (1978). *Food Processing and Nutrition.* (Academic Press, London)

Bognar, A. (1980). Nutritive value of chilled meals. In Glew, G. (ed.) *Advances in Catering Technology*, p. 387. (Applied Science Publishers Ltd., London)

Cross, G. A. and Fung, D. Y. C. (1982). *CRC Crit. Rev. Food Sci. Nutr.*, **16**, 355–81

Department of Health and Social Security (1980). *Guidelines on Precooked Chilled Foods*

Department of Health and Social Security (1984). *Diet and Cardiovascular Disease.* Report on Health and Social Subjects No. 28. (HMSO, London)

The Food Hygiene (General) Regulations (1970). (HMSO, London)

Glew, G. (1980). The contribution of large scale feeding operations to nutrition. *Wld. Rev. Nutr. Diet.*, **34**, 1–45

Glew, G., Hill, M. A. and Millross, J. (1971). Vitamins: the position now in large scale catering. In Stein (ed.) *Vitamins.* (Churchhill-Livingstone, London)

Hartley, E. and Ryley, J. (1984). The sodium content of convenience and traditionally prepared school meals. *Hum. Nutr. Appl. Nutr.*, **38A**, 60–4

Hunt, C. (1984). Nutrient losses in cook-freeze and cook-chill catering. *Hum. Nutr. Appl. Nutr.*, **38A**, 50–9

Lawson, J. M. (1982). Nutrient losses during the warmholding of food. Paper presented at the C.O.S.T. 91 Nutrition Symposium, Huddersfield, 1982

Lawson, J. M., Hunt, C. and Glew, G. (1983). Nutrition and catering. *BNF Nutr. Bull.*, **38**, 93–104

Ministry of Agriculture, Fisheries and Food (1985). *Household Food Consumption and Expenditure, 1983.* Annual Report of the National Food Survey Committee. (HMSO, London)

Ryley, J. (1981). Nutritional aspects of fast foods. *Chem. Ind.*, **14**, 497–500

Ryley, J. (1983). The impact of fast foods on UK nutrition. *Proc. IFST*, **16**, 58–64

Ryley, J. (1984). The nutritional quality of school meals from convenience foods compared with traditionally prepared dishes. *Hum. Nutr. Appl. Nutr.*, **38A**, 42–9

2
Better health through nutrition. Legislation or education?

E. M. WIDDOWSON

ABSTRACT

Legislation about food has primarily concerned rationing in times of shortages and war to ensure fair distribution of food, provision of cheap or free meals, milk and welfare foods and vitamin supplements for specially needy groups and fortification of foods with minerals and vitimins. On the whole, the aims and achievements have been good, but legislation has its limitations, and actions can be taken in wartime which would be impossible in times of peace and plenty. For example, the rationing and reduction in intake of fat and sugar and the increase in the extraction rate of flour made necessary during the Second World War are some of the measures advocated at the present time for better health through nutrition. Mandatory fortification of foods with minerals and vitamins continues today without much outcry, but no laws will stop people eating all the fat and sugar they want. In times of peace and plenty, a reduction in consumption of foods that are freely available can only be brought about by education and persuasion.

From the 1930s onwards committees were set up by various

organisations to make recommendations about health, food and nutrition. The Medical Research Council sponsored research on nutrition and the work was published as a series of reports. In the 1960s the Department of Health established its Committee on Medical Aspects of Food Policy which has set up panels and working parties over the years to consider subjects of current importance, and to report and advise thereon. The special needs of infants, children, the elderly and Asian immigrants have all been covered, as well as the nutritional aspects of bread and flour and of foods which simulate meat. Diet and cardiovascular disease has been considered by two advisory panels who reported in 1974 and 1984. The 1984 report has received wide publicity not only for its recommendations, but also for the way they are set out and the suggestions as to how they can be implemented. However, few people read scientific and medical reports; they need interpreting and their recommendations publicising, and this is one of the important functions of the British Nutrition Foundation. A booklet prepared by the British Nutrition Foundation/Health Education Council Joint Advisory Committee on Nutrition Education, shortly to be published, which interprets in practical terms the recommendations of the COMA report on Diet and Cardiovascular Disease for the housewife and caterer, is an example of education for better health through nutrition.

DISCUSSION

Legislation about nutrition goes back a long way. It has often been introduced in times of food shortage or even anticipated food shortage, and perhaps the first recorded example is when Pharaoh dreamed a dream which was interpreted by Joseph to mean that there would be seven years of plenty in Egypt, followed by seven years of famine. On Joseph's advice Pharaoh decreed that corn should be stored during the seven years of plenty to provide for the seven lean years, which apparently it did (Genesis, 41). It is a sad reflection on modern science that the present shortages in Ethiopia and the Sudan were not foreseen and provided for as they were in

Egypt thousands of years ago.

In our country when shortages have come, generally as the result of bad harvests or wars, our kings, on the advice of our Government, have also issued proclamations asking for the more well-to-do to economise on corn for the sake of the poor. Thus, as a result of the bad harvest in 1800, King George III issued a proclamation to be read in all churches on two successive Lord's Days: 'Out of Our tender Concern for the Welfare of Our People We thought fit (with the Advice of Our Privy Council) to issue this Our Royal Proclamation most earnestly exhorting and charging all those of Our loving Subjects who have the Means of procuring other Articles of Food than Corn ... to practise the greatest Economy and Frugality in the Use of every Species of Grain. And We do, for this Purpose, more particularly exhort and charge all Masters of Families to reduce the Consumption of Bread in their respective Families, by at least One-Third of the Quantity consumed in Ordinary Times ... to abstain from the Use of Flour in Pastry and, moreover, carefully to restrict the Use thereof in other Articles than Bread; And do also, in like Manner, exhort and charge all Persons who keep Horses, especially Horses for Pleasure, as far as their respective Circumstances will admit, carefully to restrict the Consumption of Oats and other Grain for the Sustenance of the Same.'

By the beginning of the First World War England depended very largely on imported grain both for the human and animal population, and the shortage created by the German submarine campaign, which started in October 1916, brought about a state of affairs comparable with the conditions which followed the bad harvests of 1800. Up to this time there had been no rationing, and in fact the Government was very much against it. What seemed to bother them particularly was a shortage of sugar. However, things got so bad and prices rose so high that something had to be done. One trouble was that, although there was a lot of information about imports and food production at home in times of peace, nobody knew what was the least amount of food energy on which people could live without coming to much harm. A committee had already been set up by the Royal Society with a panel of experts who could give advice on physiological problems arising in wartime. A new Ministry of Food was established and Lord Davenport was appointed as Food Controller. He did not believe in scientific advice, and could not understand that scientists could know more about food than one who, like himself, had spent a lifetime as a provision merchant (Drummond and Wilbraham, 1974). In February 1917 he appealed to the public for a system of voluntary rationing of bread, meat and sugar. The rations he proposed would have provided so few calories that people would have needed to eat far more of other foods such as fats and potatoes, and these were just not available. The Royal Society Committee was very critical of this, as it was of the 'Meatless Day', also introduced by Lord Davenport. Then in May 1917 things came to a head, Lord Davenport resigned and Lord Rhondda took over. As in 1800, the supply of grain was a great problem because so much was imported and again the King, George V this time, issued a proclamation to be read in churches on four successive Lord's Days. The wording was almost exactly the same as that of George III's proclamation. Even this was not enough, and in February 1918 meat, butter, margarine and sugar were rationed. Meantime 'war bread' had come in and the extraction rate of the flour had gradually risen to 92%. However, bread was never rationed.

In the Second World War the system of rationing and food distribution was completely different from the muddle of 1916–1918. There were several reasons for this. Scientific knowledge about food and nutrition had increased, we knew far more about food supplies and food requirements, and Drummond was appointed Scientific Adviser to the Ministry of Food. He was Professor of Biochemistry at University College, London. He was concerned about nutrition, and he was the ideal man for the job. He set out not only to maintain but to improve the nutrition of the nation. This he succeeded in doing, and some of the measures introduced of necessity, such as the rationing of fats and sugar and the increase in the extraction rate of flour, are what we regard today as healthy eating. Legislation about food in the Second World War was undoubtedly of great benefit to the health of the nation.

Besides regulating distribution of food by rationing in times of food shortage in wartime, legislation had been introduced over the years in peacetime and some of this has concerned particularly vulnerable or needy groups. It all started with the publication in 1900 of a book by Seebohm Rowntree called *Poverty, A Study of Town Life*. In it he described the bad conditions under which the poor were living in the city of York. This was followed some years later by a memorandum from Sir William Taylor, Director General of the Army Medical Services, in which he described the poor physique of men enlisting for service in the Boer War. An Interdepartmental Committee was appointed and one of the conclusions in its report, published in 1904, was that many women and children were living on diets very inadequate both in quantity and quality. The recommendations of the Committee led to the Education Act (Provision of Meals) which was passed in 1906. By 1911 more than 200 000 poor school children were receiving free meals. Diets in prisons also came in for criticism and led to the setting up of another Interdepartmental Committee which, with medical advice, made recommendations as to how prison diets should be improved. At the turn of the century, when all this was going on, nothing was known about vitamins, so all that was considered was energy and protein. By good fortune the diets introduced for children in institutions by the Local Government Board contained milk, three-quarters to one pint a day.

Between the wars came the depression and once again there was great poverty. The Minister of Health appointed a Panel on Nutrition. Vitamins were now regarded as all-important and the first report of the Panel stressed the necessity of protective foods such as milk, cheese, fruit and fat fish, foods which families of the unemployed could not afford.

A person who had great influence in the 1930s was Lord Boyd Orr. As reported in the Boyd Orr Lecture given to the Nutrition Society in 1983 (Widdowson, 1984), it was he who really brought home to the Government the importance of cows' milk for children and it was as a result of his studies and those of Corry Mann (1926) that in 1934 the Milk Act was passed, making milk available to children at elementary schools for ½d for one-third of a pint. Only about half the children took advantage of the scheme, probably because a halfpenny per day for a child was too much for many large families to pay. This 'Milk in Schools' scheme was to continue for the next forty years.

One disadvantage of the scheme was that it did not cater for children below school age and it was not until 1941, under the influence of Drummond, that the National Milk Scheme was introduced to provide cheap milk for pregnant women and children up to 5 years and the Vitamins Welfare Scheme to make available for them orange juice and cod-liver oil tablets containing vitamins A and D. Again people had a choice; they need not take the milk or vitamins, and many of them chose not to take their entitlement.

It is when legislation leaves no freedom of choice that problems arise, and this brings me to the mandatory fortification of food. Bread and margarine are the only two foods for general consumption that have to be fortified with nutrients to comply with the statutory regulations in this country. In 1940 Drummond submitted a memorandum to the Ministry of Food in which he recommended that margarine should be fortified with vitamins A and D. His object was to make margarine not only similar to summer butter, but also to compensate, to some extent, for the shortage of eggs, which are one of the few natural foods rich in vitamin D. Drummond's recommendations were implemented and they have never been revoked. By law, each 100 g margarine must contain 800–1000 μg of vitamin A and 7–9 μg of vitamin D. In fact, the vitamin D is about 10 times the amount naturally present in butter and even today margarine is for some people the most important dietary source of vitamin D. As far as I know, there was no outcry about this measure for, after all, people don't have to eat margarine. When it came to bread, our staple food, however, it was quite another matter.

In the early 1940s we made a long series of balance experiments on ourselves and other people in which we measured the absorption of calcium from bread made from various kinds of flour and we showed that the phytate in higher extraction flour interfered with calcium absorption. Calcium absorption was improved by adding calcium, either as carbonate or phosphate, to the flour (McCance and Widdowson, 1942). Partly as a result of these experiments, it was decided that the wartime 85% extraction flour should, by law, be fortified with calcium carbonate. The grounds for this measure were, first, that the 85% National Wheatmeal flour used for bread-making contained more phytate than pre-war white flour and, second, that owing to the severe rationing of milk and cheese, the diets of the majority of the people in Britain would not contain enough calcium to meet their requirements. This decision aroused a storm of protest. The millers said it would produce 'rope' in the flour, and long before any calcium had been added, descriptions of the harmful effects it was producing were pouring into the Ministry of Food. It was said to be causing hardening of the arteries, stones in the kidneys and various other ills. A man called Isaac Harris was particularly vociferous and he wrote a number of letters to *The Lancet*, opposing the fortification.

> 'It can be demonstrated with mathematical precision that, in the case of many middle-aged people who suffer from weakness of the kidney, the added calcium must shorten life . . . For no reason at all, millions of adults are compelled to swallow such a potent substance as calcium which they do not require and some of whom are bound to suffer hurt from it' (Harris, 1942).

Nevertheless, the addition of calcium carbonate to flour became statutory and the objections soon died down. In fact, there was one flour that was exempted from the regulations and that was wholemeal. This was in deference to the belief of the natural food enthusiasts, who wanted no chemicals added to their food. Wholemeal flour contains more phytate than any other so it, of course, needed calcium the most.

Wheat flour contains very little calcium, and in adding calcium to flour and bread we were not putting back something that milling has removed but were using our staple food as a vehicle for a nutrient we thought people needed.

Three other nutrients, iron, thiamin and nicotinic acid, have also been subject to the Flour (Composition) Regulations, but here the story is rather different. It is well known that wholemeal 100% extraction flour contains more of these constituents than white flour. Intermediate extractions, for example the 85% extraction National flour used in wartime, came in-between. For this reason, and also because Dame Harriette Chick had shown that weanling rats grew better on 100% and 85% extraction flours than on white flour with added vitamin B_1 (Chick, 1940; Chick, 1942), we believed that brown bread was a better food for men, women and children than white bread, provided that the problem about phytate in brown bread was overcome by adding calcium carbonate to it. At this time no one was interested in dietary fibre.

In 1946 there was a shortage of wheat in this country, partly because of a world shortage, and partly because the Government had 'lent' 600 000 tons of cereals to the semi-starving countries of Europe. The extraction rate was raised to 90% in May and bread began to be rationed in July. Bread rationing was an entirely new departure, wisely avoided during both World Wars, and contrary to the physiological principles laid down by the Royal Society's Committee in the First World War. It could probably have been avoided by raising the extraction rate still further, and in fact the extraction rate was brought down to 85% before rationing ended and this continued until July 1948.

In 1955 an independent panel, under the chairmanship of Lord Cohen, was set up to advise the Government on the kind of flour that should be used for bread-making in this country. The report of our studies in Germany had been published by this time, which showed that children grew and improved in health and physique just as well whether 75% of their energy came from wholemeal, 85% extraction or white bread (Widdowson and McCance, 1954). In our conclusions we were careful to say that this applied under the conditions of our experiments, and particularly in relation to the rest of the diet. The German children had very little milk, meat, fish or cheese but they did have vegetables in fairly large quantities, mostly made into soups. We gave evidence to the Cohen

Committee. Their report stated that 'The available evidence did not reveal any ascertainable difference between National — that is, 85% extraction flour — and flour of lower extraction rate to which the three nutrients had been restored, i.e., iron, thiamin and nicotinic acid, which would affect the health of the population in any foreseeable circumstances' (Panel on Composition and Nutritive Value of Flour, 1956). The panel was not willing to go back to pre-war unenriched white flour and, as a result of its recommendations, the Flour (Composition) Regulations 1956 decreed that all flour should contain not less than 1.65 mg iron, 0.24 mg thiamin and 1.6 mg nicotinic acid per 100 g. These are the amounts in 80–85% extraction flour, but it was no longer compulsory to mill to the higher extraction rate to achieve them. They could be added in the correct proportions to white flour. The iron was to be added either as ferrum redactum — reduced iron — or as ferric ammonium citrate. The millers preferred reduced iron because it did not make the flour go rancid. However, reduced iron, which is made by passing hydrogen over ferric oxide under controlled conditions, disappeared from the British pharmacopoeia about the time that it was supposed to be put into flour and it was no longer obtainable. The millers, therefore, used powdered metallic iron, and it was later shown by Elwood (1968) that powdered iron is not soluble in gastric juice, and it therefore passes through the digestive tract without being absorbed. In the Flour Regulations of 1963 and 1974 the method of manufacture of ferrum redactum is clearly specified.

On three occasions in the past twenty-five years, COMA was asked by the Food Standards Committee of the Ministry of Agriculture, Fisheries and Food to advise on the nutritional aspects of bread and flour. The Food Standards Committee is an important standing committee keeping a watchful eye on all aspects of food composition. Advisory Panels were set up by COMA and their reports were published in 1960 (MAFF), 1974 (MAFF) and 1981 (DHSS). I was a member of the two later panels. On the first occasion it was recommended that the additions of calcium, iron, thiamin and nicotinic acid should remain as they were.

The panel that met on the second occasion agreed that fortification with calcium carbonate was no longer necessary because the original reasons for adding it no longer applied. White flour containing very little phytate was used for bread-making and the calcium-rich foods, milk and cheese, were freely available. However, at the last moment it was decided to reverse this decision, largely because papers had been published by Crawford and others (Crawford and Crawford, 1967; Crawford, Gardner and Morris, 1971) suggesting that in hard water areas such as London deaths from heart disease were lower than in soft water areas like Glasgow. The recommendations in the 1974 report, however, are set out in a very negative way: 'We therefore do not recommend that chalk be no longer added to flour'.

The latest Advisory Panel appointed by COMA to consider nutritional aspects of bread and flour (DHSS, 1981) recommended, after much thought and deliberation, 'that the addition of calcium carbonate (chalk) to any flour be no longer necesary and that the restoration of iron, thiamin and nicotinic acid to flour be no longer mandatory'. This recommendation was accepted by the Ministry of Agriculture, Fisheries and Food and included in their draft regulations of April 1983. However, after this there began a campaign to try to persuade the Ministry to think again. There was a television programme and correspondence in *The Lancet* (Robinson *et al.*, 1983) foretelling the harm that would befall us, and particularly older people, if chalk were no longer added to flour — in other words, Isaac Harris in reverse. Age Concern and the correspondence columns of *The Times* became involved, as did the millers, who now wanted to keep chalk in flour just as much as in 1942 they wanted to keep it out. In the end expediency rather than science prevailed, and when the Bread and Flour regulations of 1984 were published calcium carbonate had still to be added to flour to give a concentration of 235-390 mg calcium per 100 g flour, and iron, thiamin and nicotinic acid to reach the same concentrations as before. Probably one of the main reasons behind the decision to leave everything in *status quo* was that the additions do no harm and, even if they are not necessary now, they may be at some time in the future, and it is far easier to leave things as they are now than to stop mandatory fortification and then reintroduce it.

I have gone into the story of bread in some detail because I was involved in it. I want now to say a little about research and education as a means of promoting better health through nutrition. Serious education about nutrition and health could not begin until the science of nutrition had advanced far enough to make this a worthwhile exercise. During the First World War there was much exhortation of the public about economising on food, and leaflets and booklets were distributed advising people how to do this. However, it was not very scientific, and it was only after the war ended that it was appreciated how much growth and health depended upon good nutrition, and how important scientific research was in increasing knowledge about the subject. The 1920s and 1930s saw the setting up of committees to consider various aspects of better health through nutrition. These were really the successors of the Royal Society Committee which had given such sound advice to the Government during the First World War, and whose advice was, at first, largely ignored.

The Medical Research Committee, which was established in 1913, received a Royal Charter and became the Medical Research Council in 1920. Much of the research work on nutrition in the 1920s and 1930s was sponsored by the Medical Research Council and the findings were published in the Special Report Series. These were reports of research findings, but some of them led to publicity and even to legislation. A few of the more influential ones were *Studies of Rickets in Vienna (1919–1922)* by Dame Harriette Chick and others (Chick *et al.*, 1923), *Report on the Nutrition of Miners and their Families* by the MRC Committee upon Quantitative Problems in Human Nutrition, of which Cathcart was the Chairman, which was published in 1924 (MRC), *Diets for Boys during the School Age* by Corry Mann, published in 1926, and *Poverty, Nutrition and Growth* by Paton and Findlay, also published in 1926. Most of the MRC Special Report Series are now out of print, but *The Composition of Foods* (Paul and Southgate, 1978) is still going strong and is now in its fourth edition.

In 1933 the British Medical Association appointed a committee 'to determine the minimum weekly expenditure on foodstuffs which must be incurred by families of varying size if health and working capacity are to be maintained and to construct specimen diets'. Their report, published in 1933, gives advice on diets for limited incomes and their estimated cost of an adequate diet was 5/- to 6/- per man per week. Even this amount was beyond the means of many poor families. The cause was taken up by Sir John Boyd Orr, whose book *Food, Health and Income*, published in 1936, was an important landmark in bringing to public notice the difference in diet and in state of nutrition between different economic classes.

The Second World War brought education about nutrition as well as excellent legislation. Leaflets and posters were issued advising housewives how to use the dried eggs, National Household Milk and dried skimmed milk, and lectures and demonstrations were organised by the Advice Division of the Ministry of Food. Domestic Science teachers, dietitians, school meals organisers and hospital caterers all played their part in disseminating knowledge about wartime nutrition and health. The King Edward's Hospital Fund for London published two memoranda on hospital diets, in 1943 and 1945.

One of the earlier reports issued by the Ministry of Health on the subject of nutrition was *Requirements of Man for Protein*, published in 1964. This report was essentially the evidence assembled by a Working Party under the chairmanship of Sir Frank Young for submission to the Advisory Committee on Nutrition and Food Policy of WHO and FAO. The Committee on Medical Aspects of Food Policy (COMA for short) was not then in existence, but it was set up soon afterwards. Sir George Godber, who was the Chief Medical Officer at that time, was largely instrumental in its establishment and was for many years its Chairman. It set up working parties and panels to consider various aspects of nutrition and health. Their reports are published as a series of *Grey Books*, and over the past 15–20 years have covered such subjects as *Iron in Flour* (DHSS, 1968); *Recommended Intakes of Nutrients for the United Kingdom* (DHSS, 1969 and updated in 1979); *Nutrition of the Elderly*

(DHSS, 1970); *Nutrition Survey of Pre-School Children* (DHSS, 1975); *Diet and Coronary Heart Disease* (DHSS, 1974); Artificial Feeds for the Young Infant (DHSS, 1980); *Rickets and Osteomalacia* (DHSS, 1980); *Foods which simulate Meat* (1980); *Nutritional Aspects of Bread and Flour* (DHSS, 1981), which I have already discussed, and one that has perhaps received more publicity than most, *Diet and Cardiovascular Disease*, which was published in 1984 (DHSS).

The report on *Rickets and Osteomalacia*(1980) is a good example of having to decide whether to recommend legislation or education. I was Chairman of the Working Party that prepared the report. In the late 1970s there was a strong lobby from doctors, working in cities where there were many Asian immigrants, for the compulsory fortification of chapatti flour with vitaman D. Chapatti flour is not a special flour, it is merely wheatmeal flour used for making wheatmeal bread. It would be an impossible imposition to compel millers to fortify part of their wheatmeal flour with vitamin D, and yet to prosecute them if vitamin D were found in the other part. Moreover, the women and young children who suffered from osteomalacia and rickets were not the big eaters of chapattis and, further, not all Asians eat chapattis. We discussed the possible fortification of milk or butter with vitamin D, but then all milk or butter would have to be fortified and this we were not prepared to recommend. The toxicity of an excess of vitamin D was very much in our minds. We concluded and recommended that education was the answer — teaching the Asians to expose some of their skin and that of their infants to sunshine, and to take up the vitamin supplements to which they were entitled. Our recommendations were adopted and the 'Stop Rickets Campaign' was launched. A small team moved round from one city to another with films, posters, literature and talks. This has succeeded and the problem of rickets and osteomalacia seems to have faded away.

The Royal College of Physicians has also set up committees in recent years to consider nutrition subjects. One report, published in 1981, was on *Medical Aspects of Dietary Fibre*, and another, published in 1983, on *Obesity*. In 1984 came a report prepared jointly by the Royal College of Physicians and the British Nutrition Foundation on *Food Intolerance and Food Aversion*. Besides these, an *ad hoc* committee was set up by the National Advisory Committee on Nutrition Education to prepare a discussion paper on *Proposals for Nutritional Guidelines for Health Education in Britain*. This NACNE paper was published in 1983 and received wide publicity. It was intended as a discussion document, not a set of rules to be followed, but after it was published it was taken by some as the last word in how to eat for better health. Among its long-term proposals were a reduction in intakes of fat and saturated fatty acids, sugar, salt and alcohol and an increase in dietary fibre. It also recommended fuller labelling of foods. Most of these recommendations had been set out in the Department of Health's *Eating for Health* booklet published five years before. The recommendation about dietary fibre is the one that has 'caught on', as anyone who shops for food will know. I think this is largely due to clever advertising. Manufacturers of cereal foods saw there was something in this for them, and they acted accordingly.

The COMA Panel on Diet and Cardiovascular Disease, which reported in 1984 and which was concerned with one aspect of our present-day ills, had as its remit 'to advise the Committee on Medical Aspects of Food Policy on the significance of the relation between nutrition and cardiovascular disease, and to make recommendations'. The recommendations do not contradict those of NACNE, but expand them, and particularly take into account how they can be implemented by individuals within the population. They are addressed separately to the general public, medical practitioners, health education workers, and producers, manufacturers and distributors of food and drink, and caterers. Finally, there are recommendations for further review, and recommendations to Government. This seems to be one of the most important aspects of the report for, as far as I know, it is the first COMA report to pay special consideration to all the groups of people who should act on the advice contained in it.

Most of the reports I have mentioned, produced by the MRC, COMA panels and working parties, the Royal College of Physicians and other bodies, are specialised documents not particularly appealing to the general public, and even the COMA report on *Diet and Cardiovascular Disease* is unlikely to be seen by more than a tiny proportion of the population. The reports need interpreting and the recommendations setting out in an attractive and understandable way. To this end the Department of Health has issued some excellent illustrated booklets, for instance *Vitamin D Deficiency and Osteomalacia* (1976) and *Eating for Health* (1978), which I have already mentioned.

The Health Education Council is active in disseminating information about healthy eating. The British Nutrition Foundation has as one of its main objectives the provision of sound advice, based on scientific evidence, to educate caterers, food manufacturers, professional health-care workers, teachers and housewives about how to achieve better health through nutrition. It does this through its Scientific Advisory and Industrial Scientists Committee and produces briefing papers and longer reports representing the work of task forces which consider in greater depth nutritional subjects of current concern. The British Nutrition Foundation/Health Education Council Joint Advisory Committee on Nutrition Education (JACNE) was set up in 1984 to advise both the BNF and the HEC on nutrition education. As a first priority JACNE was asked by the Councils of the BNF and HEC at the request of the Secretary of State for Social Services to turn the advice of the 1984 COMA report on *Diet and Cardiovascular Disease* into practical guidance for a sensible healthy diet for families. A booklet is being prepared which will be aimed at the ordinary members of the public. We look forward to its publication.

In conclusion, legislation and education are not alternatives. They have been, and still are both essential means of promoting better health through nutrition. In times of food shortage and poverty, legislation has been of paramount importance. In times of peace and plenty, such as we are experiencing today, when most of the emphasis is on eating less of certain foods, it is only by education that this can be brought about.

The British Nutrition Foundation is playing its part, particularly through the Joint Advisory Committee on Nutrition Education, but we look ultimately to caterers, food manufacturers, teachers, doctors and health-care workers, who deal directly with consumers, to teach them and persuade them that better health can be achieved through nutrition.

References

British Medical Association (1933). Report of Committee on Nutrition. *Br. Med. J. (Suppl.)*, 25 November 1933. (BMA, London)

Chick, H. (1940). Nutritive value of white flour with vitamin B_1 added and of wholemeal flour. *Lancet*, **ii**, 511–12

Chick, H. (1942). Biological value of the proteins contained in wheat flours. *Lancet*, **i**, 405–8

Chick, H., Dalyell, E. J., Hume, E. M., Mackay, H. M. M., Henderson-Smith, H. and Wimberger, H. (1923). *Studies of Rickets in Vienna, 1919–1922: Report of the Accessory Food Factors Committee*. MRC Special Report Series, No. 77. (HMSO, London)

Corry Mann, H. C. (1926). *Diets for Boys during the School Age*. MRC Special Report Series, No. 105. (HMSO, London)

Crawford, T. and Crawford, M. D. (1967). Prevalence and pathological changes in ischaemic heart disease in a hard-water and in a soft-water area. *Lancet*, **i**, 229–32

Crawford, M. D., Gardner, M. J. and Morris, J. N. (1971). Changes in water-hardness and local death rates. *Lancet*, **ii**, 327–9

Department of Health and Social Security (1968). *Iron in Flour*. Reports on Public Health and Medical Subjects, No. 117. (HMSO, London)

Department of Health and Social Security (1969). *Recommended Intakes of Nutrients for the United Kingdom*. Reports on Public Health and Medical Subjects, No. 120. (HMSO, London)

Department of Health and Social Security (1970). *First Report by the Panel on Nutrition of the Elderly*. Reports on Public Health and Medical Subjects, No. 123. (HMSO, London)

Department of Health and Social Security (1974). *Diet and Coronary Heart Disease.* Report on Health and Social Subjects, No. 7. (HMSO, London)

Department of Health and Social Security (1975). *A Nutrition Survey of Pre-School Children, 1967–68.* Report on Health and Social Subjects, No. 10. (HMSO, London)

Department of Health and Social Security (1976). *Vitamin D Deficiency and Osteomalacia.* Topics of our time, No. 1. (HMSO, London)

Department of Health and Social Security (1978). *Eating for Health.* (HMSO, London)

Department of Health and Social Security (1979). *Recommended Daily Amounts of Food Energy and Nutrients for Groups of People in the United Kingdom.* Report on Health and Social Subjects, No. 15. (HMSO, London)

Department of Health and Social Security (1980). *Foods which simulate Meat.* Report on Health and Social Subjects, No. 17. (HMSO, London)

Department of Health and Social Security (1980). *Artificial Feeds for the Young Infant.* Report on Health and Social Subjects, No. 18. (HMSO, London)

Department of Health and Social Security (1980). *Rickets and Osteomalacia.* Report on Health and Social Subjects, No. 19. (HMSO, London)

Department of Health and Social Security (1981). *Nutritional Aspects of Bread and Flour. Report of the Panel on Bread, Flour and other Cereal Products.* Report on Health and Social Subjects, No. 23. (HMSO, London)

Department of Health and Social Security (1984). *Diet and Cardiovascular Disease.* Report on Health and Social Subjects, No. 28. (HMSO, London)

Drummond, J. C. and Wilbraham, A. (1939). *The Englishman's Food.* (Jonathan Cope, London)

Elwood, P. C. (1968). Radioactive studies of the absorption by human subjects of various iron preparations from bread. In *Iron in Flour.* Ministry of Health Reports on Public Health and

Medical Subjects, No. 117. (HMSO, London)
Harris, I. (1942). Chalk in bread. *Lancet*, **i**, 780–1
Interdepartmental Committee on Physical Deterioration (1904). *Report*. (HMSO, London)
James, W. P. T. (1983). A discussion paper on proposals for nutritional guidelines for health education in Britain. Prepared for the National Advisory Committee on Nutrition Education. (Health Education Council, London)
McCance, R. A. and Widdowson, E. M. (1942). Mineral metabolism of healthy adults on white and brown bread dietaries. *J. Physiol.*, **101**, 44–85
Medical Research Council Committee upon Quantitative Problems in Human Nutrition (1924). *Report on the Nutrition of Miners and their Families*. MRC Special Report Series, No. 87. (HMSO, London)
Ministry of Agriculture, Fisheries and Food (1960). Report of the Joint Nutrition Panel on Bread and Flour. In *Food Standards Committee Report on Bread and Flour, Appendix III*, pp 22–36. (HMSO, London)
Ministry of Agriculture, Fisheries and Food (1974). Committee on Medical Aspects of Food Policy. Report of the Advisory Panel on Bread and Flour. In *Food Standards Committee Second Report on Bread and Flour, Appendix V*, pp 78–119. (HMSO, London)
Ministry of Health (1964). *Requirements of Man for Protein*. Report on Public Health and Medical Subjects, No. 111. (HMSO, London)
Orr, J. B. (1936). *Food, Health and Income*. (Macmillan, London)
Panel on Composition and Nutritive Value of Flour (1956). (HMSO, London)
Paton, D. N. and Findlay, L. (1926). *Poverty, Nutrition and Growth. Studies of Child Life in Cities and Rural Districts of Scotland*. MRC Special Report Series, No. 101. (HMSO, London)
Paul, A. A. and Southgate, D. A. T. (1978). *McCance and Widdowson's 'The Composition of Foods'*, 4th edn. MRC Special Report Series, No. 297. (HMSO, London)
Robinson, C. J., Appleton, D. R., Eastoe, J. E., Hackett, A. F. and

Rugg-Gunn, A. J. (1983). Bone disease and the removal of calcium fortification from flour. *Lancet*, **i**, 1340

Rowntree, B. S. (1900). *Poverty, A Study in Town Life.*

Royal College of Physicians of London (1980). *Medical Aspects of Dietary Fibre: Summary of a Report.* (Pitman Medical, Tunbridge Wells)

Royal College of Physicians of London (1983). Obesity. *J. R. Coll. Physicians, London*, **17**, 5–65

Royal College of Physicians and British Nutrition Foundation (1984). Food intolerance and food aversion. Joint Report. *J. R. Coll. Physicians, London*, **18**, 3–41

Widdowson, E. M. (1984). Milk and the newborn animal. *Proc. Nutr. Soc.*, **43**, 87–100

Widdowson, E. M. and McCance, R. A. (1954). *Studies on the Nutritive Value of Bread and on the Effect of Variations in the Extraction Rate of Flour on the Growth of Undernourished Children.* MRC Special Report Series, No. 287. (HMSO, London)

3
The effect of catering techniques on the nutritional value of food

G. GLEW, J. LAWSON AND C. HUNT

ABSTRACT

The catering industry makes an important contribution to nutrient intake in developed countries. The primary cooking techniques of roasting, grilling, boiling and frying cause changes in the nutrient content of food, as does the traditional process of keeping food hot before service. New techniques designed to overcome some of the industry's problems such as methods known as cook-freeze, cook-chill and cook-freeze-thaw also affect the nutrient content of the food served. However, control over portion size, the recipe used and the menu could have at least as important an effect as the processing techniques on the nutritional value of the food available to users of catering services. A systems approach to catering is recommended, where the main features needing control in each system (e.g., food costs, labour costs, nutrient content and so on) are weighed against each other. The nutritional outcome of a catering technique is not the only outcome which needs control but a systems approach ensures that it is not neglected.

INTRODUCTION

In 1982 the average number of meals consumed outside the home in the UK was 3.15 per head per week, of which 1.65 were midday meals (MAFF, 1984). These figures do not include meals purchased outside the home and taken home to eat. If these take-away meals are added to the total it can be seen that the quantity of food purchased as ready-to-eat or eaten outside the home will contribute significantly to the total diet. However, these average figures do not reveal certain sub-groups within the population who rely more heavily on food consumed outside the home for their nutritional needs. Such groups would include business people working away from home during weekdays and 'captive' groups within the population such as long-stay hospital patients, some school children, the inmates of prisons and members of the armed forces.

It has been estimated that there are over 300 000 catering outlets in the UK (IGD, 1983), the largest sizeable group being pubs. About one-quarter of these outlets are 'non-profit making' in the sense that they are not operated with the sole intention of making a profit. Such outlets include workers' canteens, health-care establishments, education catering and other public service operations. The remaining 75% of outlets can be regarded as in the 'profit sector' and include restaurants, hotels, pubs and clubs, and fast food take-away outlets. However, the distribution between profit and non-profit sectors in terms of meals served is different. In 1983, 59% of meals served were classed as in the profit sector and 41% in the non-profit (Gallup, 1983). Meals served in schools to children less than 11 years old were not included in this survey. Furthermore, only 8.8% of the food purchases were to pubs in 1983, whereas the National Health Service, the state education system and canteens between them purchased over 37% of the total food purchases. Hence, it can be concluded that individual outlets in the non-profit sector are much larger and serve more meals per unit of time than in the profit sector. This conclusion leads to the view that compared with the profit sector, larger quantities of food must be prepared in the non-profit sector and that cooking methods could well be different and based on larger scale equipment. But there is also evidence that the profit sector is increasing its market share at the expense of the non-profit sector as a result of, for example, factory closures and changes in education policy.

A change in the distribution of meals produced by the two sectors could influence the types of foods consumed outside the home and this dynamic situation must be kept in mind when considering the nutritional effects of eating outside the home. Because of its share of the total market and the probability that larger scale non-profit catering is of greater nutritional significance to its, often disadvantaged, consumers, this sector has received more attention than the profit sector (Glew, 1980).

PRIMARY COOKING TECHNIQUES

The main purpose in cooking food is to convert a 'raw' product into something more palatable. In general, cooking causes softening of the texture, breakdown of cell walls and potentially increases the availability of the nutrients for absorption in the gut. However, the cooking process, particularly if not controlled, can also result in irrecoverable losses of nutrients. Cooking food requires the application of heat to the food product in some way and an understanding of the processes involved gives clues to likely effects on the nutritional value of the food.

The primary physical processes which take place in food during cooking are the transfer of heat and mass. The traditional cooking methods of boiling, baking, steaming, roasting, broiling, frying and grilling are all developments from heating food by the use of an open fire. The only methods in use not directly descended from these traditional methods are microwave and induction heating. Food is a relatively poor conductor of heat and most cooking methods require the food to be heated at the surface and the heat is transferred into the product by conduction or convection. Transfer of heat to the surface of the product is effected by some intermediary transfer medium such as air, water, steam or oil. In the case of microwave heating and infra-red heating, the energy is converted into heat inside the food but even then conduction and convection take place to transfer the heat from localised areas of higher temperature to those of lower temperature. Heat transfer into food is also influenced by the shape of the product.

Another important change which takes place is the transfer of mass largely in the form of water within the product during cooking. Cooking can therefore be seen to be a very complex process with many variables.

Kirk (1985) has designated the two processes in cooking, A and B, the ratio between which controls the speed of cooking. The two processes are:

A — the rate at which heat is absorbed by the surface of the food.
B — the rate of conduction to the centre of the food.

He points out that 'Most of the existing rules of cooking can be seen as a means of controlling this ratio'. The factors which affect A are convection (where the food is surrounded by a fluid — air, combustion products, steam, water or oil) or conduction (where the food is in direct contact with a heated surface). Convection may be either natural or forced (where the fluid is moved by a fan or pump). The rate of heat transfer is usually higher when conduction methods are used. The factors which affect B depend on the rate of evaporation from the surface of the food, the temperature of the surface and the thickness of the food. The surface area to volume ratio, that is the shape of the food, is also important. Kirk (1985) also points out that mass transfer is very important during cooking as there is considerable movement of water, flavour compounds and fat during cooking. Water migrates from the centre to the surface, fat is added or lost during heating and flavour compounds migrate within the food. In addition, micronutrients migrate and can be lost to the cooking medium by leaching.

All these changes and conditions of change which take place during cooking give the characteristic colours, flavours, odours and textures to food associated with the different cooking processes, thereby changing the palatability of the foodstuff. Concurrent with

Table 3.1 Quality changes in peas at 100 °C

Parameter	*Half-life*[a] *(mins) at 100 °C*
Thiamin	788
Texture — desirable	7
Colour — undesirable	51

[a] Half-life is the time for half the change to take place.
(From Ryley, 1985)

these changes come changes in nutritional value. Fortunately, as Lund (1983) and Ryley (1985) have pointed out, the rate of heat-induced breakdown of vitamins is very much slower than other changes which occur in food. Table 3.1 shows quality changes which take place in peas at 100 °C. The rate of thiamin degradation is much slower than texture and colour change. Table 3.2 shows a comparison of the rates of chemical change which take place in food at 121 °C. Again, vitamin destruction by heat is a slow process compared with other processes taking place. However, if the rate of softening of vegetable cell walls is high in comparison to heat destruction of vitamins then loss of water-soluble vitamins will take place rapidly into the cooking medium as a concentration gradient will exist between the cooking fluid and the foodstuff and

Table 3.2 Order of magnitude of chemical processes in food at 121 °C

Reaction	D_{121}[a]
Vitamins	100–1000
Colour, texture, flavour	5–500
Enzyme inactivation	1–10
Vegetable cells	0.002–0.02
Spores	0.1–5

[a] D_{121} is the time in minutes at 121 °C for a first order response to decay by 90%.
(Adapted from Lund, 1983)

eventually between the surface of the food and the interior. Leaching by this mechanism is likely to be the major mechanism for loss of water-soluble vitamins. Because vegetables cook at different rates (Ryley, 1985) and the rates vary at different temperatures, it will be difficult to design cooking equipment to cope with the problem automatically. The art of the vegetable chef will be with us for some time. However, it is possible that in the future catering equipment of large size could be programmed to cook automatically under controlled conditions.

Denaturation of protein takes place during cooking but gross overcooking would need to take place to reduce the nutritional value of protein. During the dry heating of meat and fish by grilling or roasting the surface protein layers will suffer heat damage but the main effect of such treatment is to improve the palatability of the product by inducing Maillard-type reactions at the surface. Deleterious changes in the fat could take place at high temperatures.

Frying is a cooking process in which the heat transfer medium — the fat — becomes a part of the cooked product and whose consumption has nutritional significance. Fried products are popular with consumers partly because of the crisp texture which is imparted by the surface dehydration of the food and partly because of the flavour and mouth feel of the resultant product. New equipment has been designed to try to reduce the overall fat content of cooked food.

Apart from the obvious technique of grilling instead of frying, much work has taken place in Sweden to try to simulate crisp textures without immersion in hot fat (Bengtsson and Dagerskog, 1977; Dagerskog and Sovenfars, 1978; Skjoldebrand and Oste, 1980). Chips are a popular potato dish and it is clear that the method used for frying influences the fat content. Recent work (West, 1985) has shown that the fat uptake by chips can be significantly lowered by using a combination of steaming, dipping in oil and oven baking rather than deep fat frying in the traditional manner. Ryley *et al.* (1980) have shown for a number of products how the fat content can be controlled and that oven frying caused less fat uptake than deep fat frying.

ASSOCIATED TECHNIQUES

The two techniques of (a) warmholding and (b) cold-holding are not 'cooking' techniques, although some cooking can go on during warmholding and some change in texture can take place during freezing. The two techniques are used as an adjunct to the primary cooking techniques and also have nutritional consequences in addition to the effects of the primary cooking. The ideal catering system exists where food is cooked to order and consumed as soon as it is cooked. In many catering situations this is difficult or impossible for logistic or economic reasons. Meals on Wheels for the elderly are cooked centrally and distributed to individual homes; large-scale catering for school children, hospital patients, prisoners and many others precludes the ideal of cooking to order followed by immediate consumption. The traditional method for coping with this problem is to try to keep the food hot in the process known as warmholding, but it is well known that this process causes deterioration in sensory quality. It is possible that deleterious changes in sensory quality caused by the practice of warmholding and rising consumer expectations of quality have led, in part, to catering operations in which the food is very simple to cook and can be cooked to order, e.g., much fast food would fall into this category.

In the past 10–15 years there has been a growing interest amongst caterers in the techniques of cold-holding of food to ease production and distribution problems (Glew, 1985), and the use of pre-cooked chilled and frozen food reheated immediately before consumption has become established. The necessity for a reheating stage in a cold-holding system has implications for the quality of the food and therefore any nutritional evaluation of cold-holding must also make reference to the nutrient losses incurred during this stage.

Warmholding

Holynski *et al.* (1983) have surveyed the practice of warmholding in the catering industry. It is interesting that a practice entrenched and unique to the catering industry and with such marked effects on sensory quality has only been studied in detail during the past 20 years, with most of the work taking place in the last 10 years. Surveys of warmholding practices have shown wide variations in the methods used and a wide range of times and temperatures. Times ranged from nil to 7½ hours but it was unusual to warmhold food for more than about 4 hours. Food internal temperatures at service ranged from 29 to 93 °C. The main concern should be to ensure that warmholding temperatures are above the maximum at which microbial growth will occur. The stipulated temperature varies from one country to another but an average is in the mid-60s centigrade. In studies involving hospitals, schools and restaurants in Sweden, Karlstrom and Jonsson (1977) observed warmholding times of 5 minutes to 7½ hours and mean temperatures at service of 54–60 °C. In the USA Cremer and Chipley (1979) measured times and temperatures in transported meals for the elderly of 30 minutes to nearly 3 hours and mean temperatures at two sites of 64 and 52 °C respectively. In this country (Turner and Glew, 1982) Meals on Wheels were warmheld for 50 minutes to 3 hours 30 minutes, with mean temperatures varying from 38 to 47 °C. Recent work in restaurants (Holynski, 1985) has revealed times of 0–¾ hours and temperatures between 48 and 99 °C have been observed in different products.

Maintaining food for some hours above 65 °C will improve its microbiological quality but will accelerate deterioration of heat-labile nutrients. In general, it was found that vitamin C was less stable than thiamin, with higher losses being associated with the higher warmholding temperature. Platt, Eddy and Pellett (1963) found 36–90% loss of ascorbic acid in vegetables served in hospital due to prolonged cooking and warmholding. Analysis of Meals on Wheels showed ascorbic acid losses ranging from 31–54% between the end of cooking and the first meal served (Turner and Glew, 1982). In another study (Turner *et al.*, 1980), small ascorbic acid losses were observed, possibly due to the very low warmholding temperature during delivery. In a study of transported school meals in the USA (Head, 1974), mean losses of 19% ascorbic acid and

20% iron were found. There was no detectable loss of riboflavin, less than 2% thiamin and less than 10% calcium. These large variations in loss are probably due to variations in warmholding temperature. The equipment used for this purpose is only crudely controlled and Holynski (1985) has observed temperature variation amongst different types of warmholding equipment of 70 °C.

Laboratory experiments have been performed under controlled conditions (for example, Karlstrom *et al.*, 1977; Hansson *et al.*, 1972; Bishop *et al.*, 1975; Paulus *et al.*, 1978) but times and temperatures tend to reflect warmholding practices in different countries — Sweden and Germany used longer warmholding times than the USA. In general, there is an inverse relationship between warmholding temperatures and the retention of vitamin C and thiamin. Thiamin is more stable than vitamin C during simulated warmholding conditions and small decreases in riboflavin and nicotinic acid occurred. There appears to be negligible losses of nicotinic acid, vitamin A, carotene, essential amino-acids and essential fatty acids.

The changes in sensory quality seem to be most important and food that is unpalatable will often not be eaten, hence sensory quality has an indirect effect on nutrient intake.

Cold-holding and reheating

As already mentioned, cook-freeze and cook-chill are catering systems which have been developed and implemented in the last 15–20 years with the intention of minimising warmholding times, apart from having other advantages such as centralising skilled labour.

Basically, nutrient losses that do occur in catering operations based on cook-freeze, cook-chill and the newer system cook-freeze-thaw (where the thawing stage is controlled) are likely to occur most frequently in the two stages of heat treatment, i.e., the prime cooking and the later regeneration of the cooked and frozen or cooked and chilled food portions, although losses during storage of chilled food could be important. Figure 3.1 shows the stages of

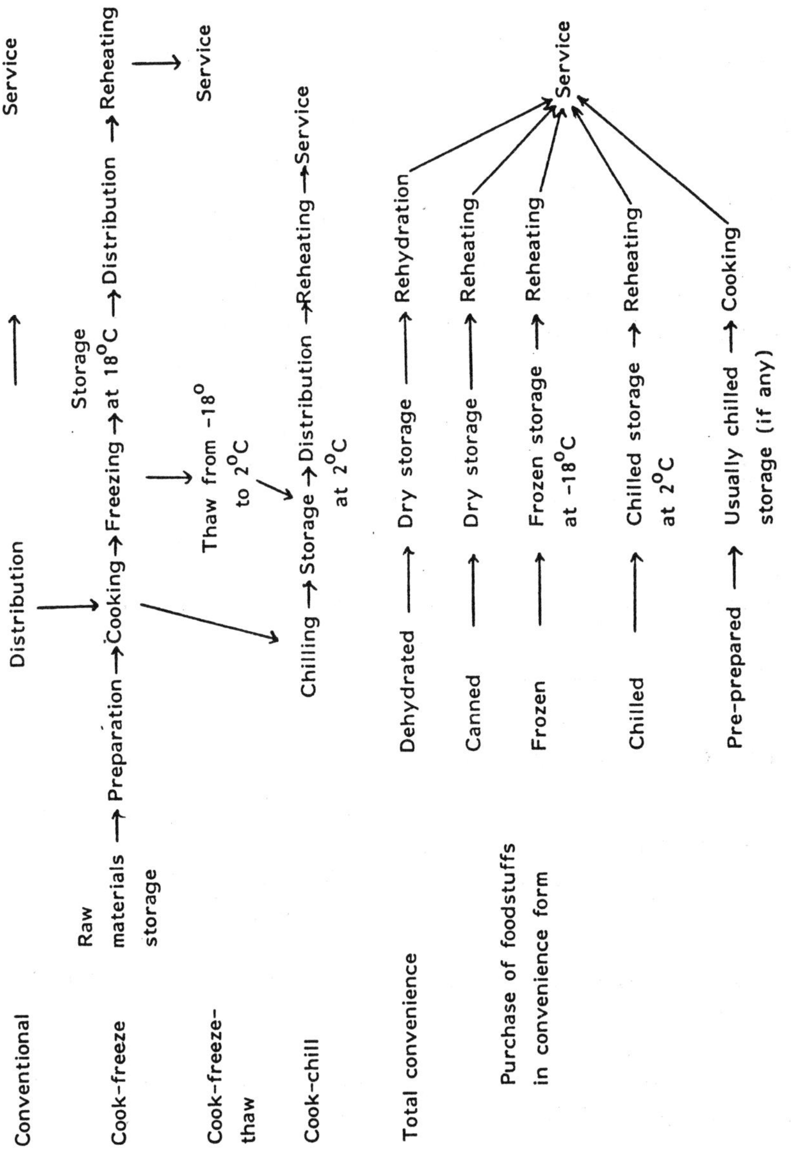

Figure 3.1 Catering systems *(From Glew, 1980)*

these new systems compared with the conventional cook-serve system.

Cook-freeze

The operation of the cook-freeze catering system has previously been adequately described (Glew, 1973), but briefly consists of centralised food preparation and cooking, portioning and blast-freezing (at an air temperature of −35 °C) during a period of up to 90 minutes. The portions are then packaged and stored frozen (at −18 °C) until required, whereupon they are transported to the site of consumption and reheated in suitable ovens.

The Catering Research Unit, set up in Leeds in 1966 and transferred in 1979 to Huddersfield Polytechnic, was largely responsible for the initial development and feasibility trials of the cook-freeze system in hospital and school meal catering (Anon., 1970; Millross *et al.*, 1973). Ascorbic acid retention in vegetables, as served, was shown to be considerably better after the introduction of cook-freeze than by the previous conventional systems which involved considerable periods of warmholding in both the hospital and school situations (Table 3.3), although the content of thiamin and riboflavin in various foods as served was reported to be generally similar when comparing the two systems.

Table 3.3 Ascorbic acid content of food served in a cook-freeze system

	Ascorbic acid content (mg/100 g)		
Catering system	*Cook-serve*	*Cook-freeze*	
Peas	1.8	12.4	Hospital[a]
New potatoes	8.6	20.3	(Glew, 1973)
Cabbage (white)	5.0	12.8	
Cauliflower	26.4	42.4	School meals[a]
Spring cabbage	18.8	26.8	(Millross *et al.*, 1973)

[a] Vitamins B_1, B_2 — similar in both systems

Considering the cook-freeze system in stages, the first factor of importance is the nutritional quality of the raw foodstuffs. An obvious example is that old potatoes tend to have a relatively low vitamin C content even in the raw state. Initial preparation of food prior to cooking can affect the nutrient content. For example, Millross *et al.* (1973), in a study of ascorbic acid loss of spring cabbage in a cook-freeze situation (which would apply equally to conventional catering), reported that over one-third of the raw content of the vitamin was lost during initial washing and shredding. Much of this loss is possibly due to enzyme action. Results from the same study also demonstrated that ascorbic acid retention after cooking decreased with increasing delay between the end of cooking and entry into the blast-freezer (Table 3.4). This is not surprising since ascorbic acid loss is known to be temperature dependent.

Table 3.4 Ascorbic acid loss in preparation of spring cabbage

1. 36% loss during initial washing and shredding (25 mins delay) before cooking

2. Delay between end of cooking and entry into blast-freezer

Delay (mins)	*% retention*[a]
18	91
25	73
55	61

[a] Freshly cooked = 100%.
(From Millross *et al.*, 1973)

There is virtually no nutrient loss during blast-freezing and relatively little loss during subsequent deep-freeze storage, since very long storage periods (i.e., several months or years) are unlikely to be used in practice in cook-freeze. Therefore, the next opportunity for significant nutrient loss is during reheating. In a properly operated cook-freeze system this reheating of food to service temperature is accomplished direct from the frozen state. However, in situations where old premises have been converted to cook-freeze, practical difficulties of equipment and transport have sometimes resulted in food being thawed in an uncontrolled way prior to reheating.

With regard to reheating direct from the frozen state, however, the dimensions of the food pack are important. Eddy *et al.* (1968) studied ascorbic acid loss during reheating of cooked/frozen potato and cabbage packs of various sizes, and concluded that the pack should have a maximum surface area and minimum practicable depth for optimal ascorbic acid retention since this allows rapid achievement of the desired internal temperature (of 70–80 °C) throughout the food. Packs of greater depth resulted in uneven heating of the food such that internal temperatures towards the surface exceeded 80 °C, resulting in precipitous vitamin C loss.

Cook-chill

An alternative to cook-freeze is the cook-chill system which is now being widely adopted. It has found some favour, partly because it is claimed to involve less recipe modification than cook-freeze, and partly because it is cheaper to install and operate. The system has previously been adequately described (Paulus *et al.*, 1980) but basically involves centralised food preparation and cooking as with cook-freeze. However, it differs thereafter, and UK Government guidelines (DHSS, 1980) recommend portioning of the food within 30 minutes of cooking followed by blast-chilling to an internal food temperature of 3 °C within a further 90 minutes. The cooked food can be stored at 0–3 °C for up to 5 days including the day of production and the day of consumption) prior to distribution. The final reheating must achieve an internal food temperature of at least 70 °C before consumption. Hence, the possible storage time of the cooked food is much less than in cook-freeze and the main hazard of cook-chill is that of microbiological safety, which can be ensured only by careful operation of the system.

In one study (Bognar, 1980), ascorbic acid loss at various stages of the cook-chill system was studied. With regard to the process of chilling, the speed of chilling of the hot cooked food down to an internal temperature of 15 °C significantly affected ascorbic acid

Table 3.5 Ascorbic acid loss linearly related to speed of chilling from an internal temperature of 80 °C to 15 °C

	Loss of ascorbic acid/hour of chilling time (%)
Mashed potato	8.5
Boiled potato	6.7
Brussel sprouts	5.0
Spinach	4.1

(From Bognar, 1980)

retention. Regression analysis yielded the results shown in Table 3.5, so that, for example, for every extra hour that it took to chill mashed potato down to 15 °C another 8.5% loss of ascorbic acid occurred. It is clear that rapid chilling is desirable and hence the use of a blast-chiller is advantageous. This ascorbic acid loss can be reduced further by chilling in a nitrogen atmosphere. Loss of other nutrients during chilling was small and there was only 10% thiamin loss with a chilling time of 5 hours.

Once the food is chilled, the next consideration is the effect of length of chilled storage (at 0–3 °C) on nutrient retention since the guidelines allow up to 5 days storage.

Results from Bognar's study suggested substantial losses of ascorbic acid, though with considerable variation between different vegetables in this respect. However, other nutrients were much less affected during chilled storage. There was no loss of retinol and small losses of thiamin and riboflavin averaging 1.9% per day for various food items (with the highest loss being for thiamin in roast pork at 4.4% per day).

Finally, the chilled food has to be reheated for service and once again ascorbic acid is the nutrient most susceptible to further loss, which is considerable. But it is interesting to note that using food portions of smaller dimensions substantially reduces ascorbic acid loss (Bognar, 1980), a finding which agrees with that of Eddy *et al.* (1968) mentioned previously. So there would appear to be relatively poor ascorbic acid retention through the cook-chill system,

Table 3.6 Ascorbic acid retention in two samples of cook-chill school meals

		Chilled		*Regeneration*	
		Retention[b] (%)	*Amount* (mg/100 g)	*Retention*[b] (%)	*Amount* (mg/100 g)
White cabbage	(4d)[a]	38	10.4	21	5.5
Chipped potatoes	(4d)[a]	37	5.8	37	5.8
Carrot/Swede	(4d)[a]	59	4.2	31	2.2
Peas	(5d)[a]	69	6.1	45	4.0
Roast potatoes	(4d)[a]	12	1.3	7	0.7
Mashed potato	(5d)[a]	32	7.8	23	5.6
Braised liver	(5d)[a]	41	4.0	41	4.0

[a] 4d = 4 days; 5d = 5 days chilled storage.
[b] Freshed cooked item = 100% retention.
(From Turner and Brown, 1981)

which makes the findings of Turner and Brown (1981) (Table 3.6) hardly surprising.

They analysed food samples for ascorbic acid taken from a cook-chill system which is in actual operation providing school meals in an area of the UK. These results show poor retention in the food, as served, after 4 or 5 days chilled storage. Similarly poor retention of ascorbic acid in vegetables as served (Table 3.7) has been observed in a recent study of cook-chill food served in hospitals (Mottishaw, 1984).

Table 3.7 Ascorbic acid content of samples at service in hospitals

	Conventional[a]	*Cook-freeze*[a]	*Cook-chill*[a]
Cabbage	4.9 (46%)	4.6 (51%)	5.7 (49%)
New potatoes	—	10.1 (74%)	15.2 (78%)
Creamed potatoes (instant)	20.1 (84%)	—	—
Chipped potatoes	2.8 (47%)	11.2 (63%)	—

[a] Ascorbic acid content (mg) per 100 g food. Percentage retention compared with freshly cooked shown in brackets.

Cook-freeze-thaw

This is a modification of the cook-freeze system which involves thawing the frozen food under controlled temperature conditions in a specially designed thaw cabinet prior to the final reheating stage. The inclusion of the thaw stage widens the potential application of the system since the use of microwaves then becomes a feasible alternative for reheating the food (Armstrong *et al.*, 1980). A further advantage of this system is that after thawing the multi-portion packs of food, portioning and plating can take place in chilled conditions. The meals can then be transported in refrigerated trolleys to distant service sites where subsequent reheating can take place. This practice should have benefits over the alternative approach of reheating frozen multi-portion packs of food in the central kitchen, plating the food whilst hot and transporting it to the service sites in heated or insulated containers.

Only limited data are available on the nutritional quality of cook-freeze-thaw meals. The results of a survey (Mottishaw, 1983), comparing losses of ascorbic acid from vegetables in a pilot cook-freeze-thaw system with those in a conventional system, are shown in Table 3.8. In the former system the mean percentage ascorbic acid retention ranged from 42% in cabbage to 82% in creamed potatoes which had been fortified with vitamin C and contained antioxidants. The percentage retention of ascorbic acid in the two systems was similar in three of the four vegetables studied, but

Table 3.8 Comparison of mean percentage ascorbic acid retention in conventional and cook-freeze-thaw catering systems

	Conventional[a]	*Cook-freeze-thaw*[a]
Cabbage	45%	42%
Peas	50%	53%
Creamed potatoes	85%	82%
Chipped potatoes	47%	56%

[a] % just cooked value present at 'consumption' stage

chipped potatoes had a higher retention rate for vitamin C in the cook-freeze-thaw system.

In summary, therefore, the data available on nutrient losses in cold-holding catering systems are limited. Nevertheless, they suggest that nutrient retention in cook-freeze systems operated with the appropriate care at each stage appears to be generally better than in a traditional system involving signficant warmholding periods.

Of the nutrients studied, cook-chill, properly operated, does not appear to involve large losses compared with freshly cooked food, except for vitamin C. With regard to this nutrient, therefore, it might be prudent to supplement a cook-chilled meal with fruit juice and/or use fortified vegetable products (e.g., mashed potato) in order to ensure a significant intake (e.g., in school meals). It is possible that losses of other labile nutrients, not yet studied, (e.g., vitamin B_6, folic acid) might be significant in cook-chill. Cook-freeze-thaw, as a catering system, could have operational advantages in some circumstances and losses will be similar to those with cook-chill, depending on the time elapsing between thawing and consumption.

CONTROL AS A DETERMINANT OF NUTRITIONAL QUALITY

A number of procedures have been discussed which can affect the nutrient content of foods provided by caterers. Many components of our diet, now considered to have importance, are unlikely to be much changed by catering procedures. Such substances would include fibre and minerals (except that the latter may be leached out).

The major determinants of nutrient content will be the quality of the foodstuffs used by caterers, the recipes they use and the portion sizes they provide. The menu from which the consumers choose their food will also affect the intake by consumers. Control by the caterer over these matters is as important as controlling times and temperatures during the processing of the food.

It is likely that caterers will attempt to purchase the freshest food available or food that is known to be relatively stable, such as the many canned, frozen and dehydrated products from the food manufacturing industry. If it is then stored under appropriate conditions, deterioration will be minimised.

The recipes that caterers use will clearly have a major effect on the nutrient content of the prepared or cooked dish. In this area there is room for considerable development in producing new or altered dishes with, for example, higher fibre, lower fat and salt and any other modification considered desirable. Such changes in the formulation of dishes could have a far greater impact on nutrient intake than some of the processing difficulties already described. In recent surveys it has been observed that commercial up-market restaurants can be providing more than 50% of the calories available in a meal as fat (Collison, 1985). Even in school meals the proportion of calories as fat was about 44%. Changes in the type of dish being offered could alter this situation markedly. The supplementation of meals with micronutrients for special groups such as the elderly could possibly be justified but little work has been done on this subject.

Portion sizes are usually related in the minds of caterers with costs. Equally, the portion sizes available also affect the total nutrient intake derived from a meal. Finally, the menu from which the consumer chooses (that is, the way in which the food is marketed) will also affect the final nutritional outcome.

Nutritional information on the nutrient content of raw food, the effects of processing techniques, including warmholding and coldholding, and possible recipe modification are all pieces of management information which the caterer has to assimilate. Management information regarding costs, the market situation, labour availability and its degree of skill, and consumer wants (as opposed to needs) are among the many factors that the caterer must weigh and evaluate during the management process. Many factors could lead to a caterer using a system which results in an end product low in some particular nutrient. Provided that he knows about the likelihood of this happening, then some corrective action can be taken possibly elsewhere in the system. Ascorbic acid may be lost for some good processing reason; recipes and menus can be adapted to correct this problem. The biggest problem is likely to be ignorance which results in failure to appreciate that a problem exists. Hence a 'systems' approach to catering can be of great relevance (Collison and Johnson, 1980) and result in control by the caterer over all aspects of his operation.

SUMMARY

The catering industry is very diverse and makes a significant contribution to food intake in developed countries and therefore needs to consider the impact of the food it provides on the nutritional intake of consumers. Primary cooking techniques cause changes in the nutrient content of food, as does the traditional process of keeping food hot before service. Newer techniques, designed to overcome some of the industry's problems, such as cook-freeze, cook-chill and cook-freeze-thaw, also have an effect on the nutrient content of food. However, control over the portion size, the recipe and careful design of the menu could have at least as important an effect as the processing techniques on the nutritional status of the caterer's end product. A systems approach to catering management is recommended, in which the main features needing control in each system (e.g., costs, labour management, nutrient content and so on) are weighed against the possible effects on other elements of the system also needing control. The nutritional outcome of a catering technique is not the only outcome which needs to be controlled but a systems approach helps to ensure that important features are not forgotten and enables corrective action to be taken.

References

Anon. (1970). *An Experiment in Hospital Catering using the Cook-Freeze System.* (University of Leeds and United Leeds Hospitals, Leeds)

Armstrong, J. F. *et al.* (1980). *The Housebound Elderly: Technical Innovations in Food Service.* (Catering Research Unit, The Polytechnic, Huddersfield)

Bengtsson, N. and Dagerskog, M. (1977). Double-sided contact heating and infra-red heating for frying foods. In Glew, G. (ed.) *Catering Equipment and Systems Design*, p. 377. (Applied Science Publishers Ltd., London)

Bishop, K., Armstrong, J. F. and Glew, G. (1975). *Some Preliminary Investigations on an insulated Food Service Tray*. Report 52. (Hotel and Catering Research Centre, Hudddersfield Polytechnic)

Bognar, A. (1980). Nutritive value of chilled meals. In Glew, G. (ed.) *Advances in Catering Technology*, p. 387. (Applied Science Publishers Ltd., London)

Collison, R. (1985). Personal communication

Collison, R. and Johnson, K. (1980). A general systems theory approach to catering. In Glew, G. (ed.) *Advances in Catering Technology*, p. 327. (Applied Science Publishers Ltd., London)

Cremer, M. L. and Chipley, J. R. (1979). Time and temperature, microbiological and sensory quality of meat loaf in a commissary food service system transporting heated food. *J. Food Sci.*, **44**, 2

Dagerskog, M. and Sorenfors, P. (1978). A comparison between four different methods of frying meat patties. *Lebensm-Wiss. Technol.*, **II**, 306 and 312

Eddy, T. P., Nicholson, A. L. and Wheeler, E. F. (1968). Precooked frozen foods: the effects of heating on vitamin C. *Nutrition*, **XXII**, 3, 123–8

Gallup (1983). Trends in catering. Presented at the *Symposium on Long Term Demands for Food in the UK.* (Agricultural Economics Society, London)

Glew, G. (ed.) (1973). *Cook-Freeze Catering: an Introduction to its Technology*. (Faber and Faber, London)

Glew, G. (1980). The contribution of large-scale feeding operations to nutrition. *Wld. Rev. Nutr. Diet*, **34**, 1

Glew, G. (1985). Refrigeration and the Catering Industry. *Proc. Inst. R. 1984–85*, **6-1**

Hansson, E., Olsson, H., Bosund, I. and Rasmussen, I. (1972).

Changes during warmholding of food products. *Naringsforskning*, **16**, 106

Head, M. K. (1974). Nutrient losses in institutional food handling. *J. Am. Diet. Ass.*, **65**, 423

Holynski, E. W., Aukland, J. N. and Glew, G. (1983). A review of the literature concerning warmholding of foods in catering. In Zeuthen *et al.* (eds) *Thermal Processing and Quality of Foods*, p. 403. (Elsevier Applied Science Publishers Ltd., London)

Holynski, E. W. (1985). Personal communication

IGD, Institute of Grocery Distribution (1983). *Catering — Serving a Service.* Report by Marketpower Ltd., London

Karlstrom, B. and Johnson, L. (1977). Quality changes during warmholding of foods. In Glew, G. (ed.) *Catering Equipment and Systems Design*, p. 315. (Applied Science Publishers Ltd., London

Karlstrom, B., Lundren, B. and Johsson, L. (1977). *Warmholding of Potatoes.* SIK Report No. 417. (Sweden)

Kirk, D. (1985). Cooking — understanding what happens in catering equipment. In Glew, G. (ed.) *Advances in Catering Technology — Three.* (Elsevier Applied Science Publishers Ltd., London)

Lund, D. B. (1983). Impact of industrial cooking of foods on its nutritional and quality characteristics. In Zeuthen, P. (ed.) *Thermal Processing and Quality of Foods*, p. 291. (Elsevier Applied Science Publishers Ltd., London)

Millross, J., Speht, A., Holdsworth, K. and Glew, G. (1973). *The Utilisation of the Cook-Freeze Catering System for School Meals.* (Catering Research Unit, University of Leeds)

Ministry of Agriculture, Fisheries and Food (1984). *Household Food Consumption and Expenditure in the UK in 1982. National Food Survey.* (HMSO, London)

Mottishaw, J. (1983). *Ascorbic Acid Content of Vegetables from a Conventional Catering System and from a Cook-Freeze-Thaw Catering Hospital System.* Laboratory Report No. 180. (Hotel and Catering Research Centre, Huddersfield Polytechnic)

Paulus, K., Nowark, J., Zacharias, R. and Bognar, A. (1978). Influence of heating and keeping warm on the quality of meals.

Ann. Nutr. Alim., **32**, 447
Platt, B. S., Eddy, T. P. and Pellett, P. L. (1963). *Food in Hospitals.* (Oxford University Press, London)
Ryley, J., Kleszko, K. and Turner, M. (1980). Fat absorption during frying. In Glew, G. (ed.) *Advances in Catering Technology*, p. 431. (Applied Science Publishers Ltd., London)
Ryley, J. (1985). The scientific basis of cooking. In Glew, G. (ed.) *Advances in Catering Technology — Three.* (Elsevier Applied Science Publishers Ltd., London)
Skjoldebrand, C. and Oste, R. (1980). Reheating of minced meat products in a convection oven. In Glew, G. (ed.) *Advances in Catering Technology*, p. 232. (Applied Science Publishers Ltd., London)
Turner, M., Ryley, J. and Kerwin, M. (1980). The nutrient content of Meals on Wheels in Leeds. In Glew, G. (ed.) *Advances in Catering Technology*, p. 284. (Applied Science Publishers Ltd., London)
Turner, M. and Brown, J. (1981). Unpublished observations
Turner, M. and Glew, G. (1982). Home delivered meals for the elderly — a nutritional study. *Food Technol.*, July, 46
West, A. (1985). Personal communication

4
Trends in eating out

G. HEALD

ABSTRACT

The average number of meal occasions per week of food purchases outside the home has been declining at the rate of about 1½% per year over the last decade. This is primarily because of the decline in factory and school meals. The commercial sector of catering has been growing at a rate of about ¾% per year. The only sector to show any real growth is take-away, which in 1984 accounted for 27% of all meal occasions compared with 14% in 1975. It also accounts for 21% of all expenditure. Amongst the lower social classes one in three purchase a take-away meal and eat it at home at least once a week, much of this being associated with watching videos.

In spite of people being bombarded with facts about healthy diet, chip potatoes are still as popular as ever and are included with 30% of all meals. Soup is still the most popular form of starter and the most popular desserts are cakes and gateaux. Britain's favourite lunch is soup, fish and chips, peas, ice-cream and coffee. Britain's favourite dinner is prawn cocktail, steak, chips and peas, gateaux and wine.

In a survey of young adults aged 15–25, which Gallup conducted for MAFF, it is shown that one in three of young women claim that they are overweight compared with 19% of young men, and this leads to great concern about what they eat. In spite of this, one in three women eat chocolate, sugar and confectionery daily. Men are much more likely to have a cooked lunch and evening meal than women. Half of teenagers read food labels and are particularly concerned about colouring, additives and preservatives in food. Liver is the most disliked food which they feel they ought to eat, followed by greens. 5% claim to have a food allergy.

TRENDS IN CATERING

This chapter examines trends in catering from both the consumer's and the caterer's point of view.

Consumer data are taken from a continuous Gallup study entitled *The British Survey of Eating Out* over the last decade, 1974–1984. Estimates of the number of meal occasions, average weekly expenditure, number of people eating out, food consumer, type of outlet and reasons for eating out are based on a diary distributed to a random sample of about 4250 individuals a year, which yields data on about 7000 meal occasions a year.

The caterer's perception of trends is based on an annual Gallup *Menu and Business Survey*, based on about 850 personal interviews in a wide range of catering establishments and conducted on behalf of the publication *Caterer and Hotelkeeper.*

CONSUMER TRENDS

Perhaps the most noticeable factor is that the overall catering market, based on the average number of meal occasions per week of food purchased outside the home, has been declining at the rate of about 1.5% a year over the last decade in spite of the introduction of some fairly sophisticated marketing operations. This does not mean that growth has been stagnant in all sectors of the catering market. In particular, the commercial sector of catering has been growing at a rate of about ¾% a year, but this has been more than offset by the decline in meals at the place of work (about 5% a year) and the decline in school meals (about 4% a year).

Table 4.1 Average number of meal occasions (per week in millions)

	Total market	*Purely commercial*	*Place of work*	*School sector* (age 11+)
1975	85.2	41.5	34.3	9.4
1984	71.2	44.6	18.1	5.4
Change over 10 years	−16%	+7%	−47%	−43%

(Source: *British Survey of Eating Out*)

These results are illustrated in Table 4.1, which shows that for the years 1975–1984 (where complete annual data are available for each year) the physical volume of meal occasions has declined by 16% over the 10-year period. In the purely commercial sector meal occasions have increased by 7%, but at the place of work there has been a massive 47% decline, and a sharp decline, of 43%, has also been registered in school meals for children aged 11 and over.

These results must be worrying for the catering industry, especially in the light of some fairly major investment programmes in certain sectors of the commercial market. Whether these investments will change British tastes in eating out, generate new demand and ultimately justify the investment must be a key question to be addressed here.

So far we have considered the trends in meal occasions away from home but how has expenditure increased over the comparable period? Are there fewer or more people eating out these days? Again, taking data from *The British Survey of Eating Out* (Table 4.2),

Table 4.2 Average expenditure amongst respondents eating out (million pounds per week)

	Total market	*Purely commercial*	*Place of work*	*School sector* (age 11+)
1975	30.4	22.4	6.6	1.4
1984	82.2	69.7	7.1	2.4
Change over 10 years	+170%	+211%	+8%	+71%

(Source: *British Survey of Eating Out*)

it can be seen that overall the market has grown by 170% in terms of expenditure over a 10-year period. In the purely commercial sector expenditure has more than kept pace with inflation, with a 211% growth. This must be compared with a growth in expenditure terms of only 8% at the place of work.

The school sector, which has recently witnessed some fairly dramatic price increases, has grown by 71% over the comparable period (1975–1984), in spite of a 43% decline in volume. Inflation for this period was 150%.

Table 4.3 shows the number of people eating out at least once a week over the comparable period.

Table 4.3 Number of people eating out at least once a week in the total market and individual segments of the market (millions a week)

	Total market	*Purely commercial*	*Place of work*	*School sector* (age 11+)
1975	22.2	17.2	7.8	2.5
1984	23.5	20.0	4.7	1.7
Change over 10 years	+6%	+16%	−40%	−32%

(Source: *British Survey of Eating Out*)

In the commercial sector, the number of people eating out at least once a week has grown by 16% to 20.0 million people a week in 1984. However, the number of people eating out at least once a week at their place of work has declined by 40% and by 32% in the school sector.

It should be noted that the individual sectors overadd compared to the total market because individuals can eat out at least once in any of the three different sectors.

From this preliminary analysis, the following conclusions can be made:

(1) The only sector to show any real growth is the purely commercial sector, where the number of people eating out has grown by 16%, the number of meals out by 7%, and

expenditure by 170% — significantly ahead of inflation, over the period 1975–1984.

This analysis suggests that the commercial market has indeed generated additional customers, mainly at the expense of the place of work, but people are eating fewer meals per head per week out of the home. Later, analysis will show that much of this growth was initially spurred on by Government legislation in the form of VAT, which gave take-away outlets a price differential over other forms of outlets. However, this advantage was removed in 1984.

(2) The place of work sector has experienced a fairly dramatic decline over this period. What factors have caused this decline? Unemployment has obviously played a major role but the decline was already taking place in the mid 70s when unemployment was relatively low. More fundamental is the structural change taking place in British industry, with heavy engineering and large plants with their incorporated canteens declining dramatically over the last decade and office workers taking their place — often with no canteen but the personnel buying take-away meals or going to the pub instead.

(3) Two factors have influenced the decline in school meals: the drop in the school population and the dramatic increase in prices as central Government and local authorities try to reduce their school meals subsidy. In fact, the study indicates that the school market has been more resilient than the place of work.

MARKET SECTOR SIZE AND RELATIVE GROWTH OR DECLINE

Having examined the overall market, it is important to identify the sectors which have grown or declined over the last decade.

Firstly, the market shares in terms of both meal occasions and

Table 4.4 Market share

	Purely commercial	*Place of work*	*School sector* (age 11+)
Meal occasions 1975	49	40	11
Meal occasions 1984	63	25	8
Expenditure 1975	73	22	5
Expenditure 1984	85	9	3

expenditure for the three principal sectors for the period 1975–1984 are shown in Table 4.4.

It can be seen that the commercial sector has increased its share of the overall market by a dramatic 14% in meal occasions and 12% in expenditure terms almost solely at the expense of the place of work sector. Generally, school meals have held their own rather better in what has been a declining market.

More important are the relative changes that have occurred within the commercial market and these are illustrated in Table 4.5 for the five different sectors which comprise the commercial sector.

Table 4.5 Shares of the total catering market for different sub-sectors of the commercial sector

	Meal occasions		*Expenditure*	
	1975	*1984*	*1975*	*1984*
Hotels, general restaurants and steak houses, carveries	10	11	29	32
Pubs, pub restaurants, clubs and places of entertainment, wine bars	9	11	16	16
Cafes, snack bars, Wimpy/McDonald type outlets/Pizza type	13	11	13	12
Take-aways, including fish and chips, bakers' shops and Kentucky Fried Chicken outlets	14	27	12	21
Store restaurants	3	3	3	4
Total commercial sector share	49	63	73	85

It can be seen that in terms of meal occasions the overall growth of the commercial sector from 49% to 65% of the overall catering market can be almost uniquely attributed to the growth in take-away meals. Included in this category are fish and chip shops, bakers' shops (which supply the large office sandwich market), the Kentucky Fried Chicken type of establishments and other, almost exclusively take-away, outlets.

The Gallup diary may underestimate the take-away market because take-away meals from a McDonalds type establishment are classified under McDonalds rather than take-away. For historical reasons, McDonalds outlets are classified as a Wimpy/McDonalds Hamburger type establishment and are included with cafes and snack bars because this was their most appropriate classification when the study commenced in 1974. However, the broad categories in Table 4.5 are further refined in the text of the report and the growth of these types of establishments is monitored carefully.

Hotels, general restaurants and steak houses have increased their market share by 1% over this period in terms of meal occasions and by 4% in expenditure terms. This is quite a creditable feat when generally the market has been 'trading down' over this period and suggests that there is still a demand for quality eating out.

Pubs and pub restaurants and places of entertainment have increased 2% over this period, in terms of meal occasions, but have remained stationary in terms of expenditure, indicating a lower expenditure per meal occasion over time. In 1978 and 1979 this category of outlets had gained 3 or 4% more of the market. More recently, renewed interest by major brewery groups and their increasing control of pub catering (which was previously the landlady's prerogative) would lead one to expect a greater increase in this sector.

Whilst McDonalds have made vast inroads into British cuisine, they still only represent a small sector of the market because their number of outlets is limited and their location is rather regionalised.

Whilst take-aways have increased their market share from 14% to 27% in terms of meal occasions, their increase in terms of expenditure has been less dramatic — from 12% to 21% — because their price rises have not been so spectacular as in other sectors. Obviously, no VAT was a factor in this period, but since it has been introduced people are turning to take-aways to provide them with their main meal of the day.

The latest Gallup research indicated that 27% of all meal occasions are take-away, that is, not consumed at the place obtained, and that just under one in three of the population of eaters out have a take-away in their home each week (Table 4.6)

Table 4.6 Is the meal consumed where obtained?

	Meal occasions (%)	*People eating out in different ways at least once a week* (%)
Consumed where obtained	71	75
Eaten at home	12	29
Eaten elsewhere	16	24

For example, in Table 4.6 12% of all meals purchased outside the home are actually consumed in the home and another 16% are consumed elsewhere, often the office or shop floor or even in the street or park. Because respondents can have a variety of different consumption patterns, the 'persons eating out' in different categories in Table 4.6 add to over 100%.

Eating take-away meals at home is particularly related to social class, as can be seen in Table 4.7.

Table 4.7 Percentage of people in different social class groups eating a take-away meal at home at least once a week

Social class	*Percentage*
AB (Professional and managerial)	16
C1 (White collar)	31
C2 (Blue collar)	34
DE (Unskilled, OAPs)	30

Clearly, the price differential of take-away meals must be an important factor influencing the lower social classes bringing in meals to their homes. Coupled with the growth in video recorders, eating fish and chips or a Chinese meal around the television has created an alternative to eating out, namely, eating in.

CONSUMPTION PATTERNS OF MEALS

How obstinate is the British palate? How much impact has Egon Ronay made on the average British meal?

Consider the following facts based on an analysis of about 7000 meal occasions for the period January to December 1984.

- 30% of all meal occasions include chipped potatoes. In the commercial sector and school sectors this rises to 47% but is only 18% at place of work.
- Soup is the most popular form of starter and is drunk at 6% of all meal occasions.
- Steak/beef accounts for 5% of all meal occasions, whereas lamb and veal account for only 2% and 1% respectively.
- Sausages, bacon and ham account for 11% of all meal occasions but in schools they account for 19% of all meals.
- Mixed dishes such as Lancashire hot pot, shepherd's pie, etc., are more popular at 6% of all meals than hamburgers (4%).

Table 4.8 Consumption patterns of meals in 1984 (based on meal occasions)

Type of meal	*Total* (%)	*Purely commercial* (%)	*Place of work* (%)	*School sector* (age 11+) (%)
Snack	52	53	52	42
Main meal	48	47	48	58
Main meal was:				
Hot	68	74	55	76
Cold	32	26	45	24

- Poultry is very popular at 5% of all meals but is hardly ever served in schools (2%).
- Fish is the most popular item and accounts for 11% of all meal occasions.
- Pizzas account for only 2% of all meals but are more popular in schools (6%).
- Chinese meals account for 3% of all commercial meals but Indian meals for only 2%.

Table 4.9 Consumption patterns of meals in 1984 (based on meal occasions)

	Total (%)	*Purely commercial* (%)	*Place of work* (%)	*School sector* (age 11+) (%)
Starter				
Soup	6	7	6	3
Fruit juice	4	4	3	4
Other	4	5	1	1
Constituent of main meal				
Lamb	2	1	2	1
Veal	1	1	1	1
Steak/beef	5	5	4	1
Pork, except bacon	3	2	4	7
Sausages, bacon, ham	11	9	16	19
Hamburger	4	5	2	3
Mixed dish	6	5	8	7
Poultry	5	6	3	2
Fish, shellfish	11	14	5	4
Egg dish	6	5	10	2
Pizza	2	2	1	6
Indian	2	2	2	2
Chinese	3	5	<1	<1
Salad	5	3	7	5
Other	1	1	2	1
Potatoes, chipped	30	33	18	47
Potatoes, roast, mashed, sauté, boiled	10	10	12	11
Snack only	52	53	52	42

Table 4.10 Consumption patterns of meals in 1984 (based on meal occasions)

	Total (%)	*Purely commercial* (%)	*Place of work* (%)	*School sector* (age 11+) (%)
Dessert				
Custard	3	1	7	11
Fresh cream	2	3	1	<1
Cooked puddings/pies	5	3	8	10
Trifle/blancmange/jelly	2	1	4	2
Mousse/whisks/whips	1	<1	1	1
Ice-cream	4	4	3	7
Cakes/pastries/gateaux	8	8	5	17
Fruit salad	1	1	1	2
Fresh fruit	3	2	6	5
Cheese	1	1	1	3
Other dessert	2	2	3	1
Nothing	74	79	71	54

- The most popular desserts are cakes and gateaux (8%), closely followed by cooked puddings and pies (6%).
- Tea is slightly more popular (24%) than coffee (21%), pri-

Table 4.11 What, if anything, to drink?

	Total (%)	*Purely commercial* (%)	*Place of work* (%)	*School sector* (age 11+) (%)
Tea	24	20	36	9
Coffee	21	20	27	9
Milk	4	3	5	11
Soft drink, fizzy	8	9	3	14
Soft drink, non-fizzy	5	3	4	19
Other non-alcoholic	3	2	3	18
Wine	5	7	1	1
Beer, ale, lager	7	10	2	1
Spirits	2	3	1	<1
Other alcoholic	1	2	1	<1
Nothing	28	32	19	24

marily because it is much more popular at the work place.

- Almost one in seven school meals (14%) includes a soft fizzy drink.
- Beer is the most popular drink — 10% of all commercial meal occasions compared to 7% for wine. This contradicts the Gallup menu survey of caterers which suggested that wine was the most popular.

Overall, these results add up to a fairly conservative consumption pattern. This picture will now be compared with those of the caterers survey, which shows that:

- Britain's favourite lunch is soup, fish and chips, peas, ice-cream and coffee.
- Britain's favourite dinner is prawn cocktail, steak, chips and peas, gateaux and wine.
- Tomato soup is the country's most popular soup but prawn cocktail is the most popular starter.
- Hamburgers are the country's best selling non-prime meat entrée.
- Cod is the most popular fish, mainly due to its use in fish and chip shops.
- Chipped potatoes are the most popular main course accompaniment.
- Peas are the most popular vegetable.
- Fruit pie is the most popular dessert, followed by ice-cream and Black Forest gateaux.

ATTITUDES TOWARDS DIET AND ITS INFLUENCE ON THE LIFESTYLE OF YOUNG PEOPLE

In 1982, Gallup was commissioned by the Ministry of Agriculture, Fisheries and Food to carry out a survey amongst a nationally representative sample of 15–25 year olds. The survey consisted of a series of group discussions (qualitative research) followed by a quantitative phase consisting of interviewing 913 respondents with a 30-minute attitude questionnaire. Each respondent was then left a

70-page diary, fully pre-coded, asking for details of all food and drink consumed either inside or outside the home during 14 consecutive days. There was a 91% response rate to the diary exercise. Respondents were asked to estimate the quantity of every item of food and drink, using household measures such as servings, portions and tablespoons.

The nutritional value of their diets was computed using McCance and Widdowson's *The Composition of Foods*, and a series of standard weights generated by MAFF was applied where necessary to the portions recorded. In summary, the survey was able to relate attitudes to food and diet to behaviour measured in terms of estimated food intake.

Perception of weight and its effect on diet

The survey reveals in Table 4.12 that 25% of young people rate themselves as being overweight, but this view is much more prevalent amongst young women (31%) than amongst young men (19%).

Table 4.12 Perception of weight

	Total (502) (%)	*Men (249)* (%)	*Women (253)* (%)
Overweight	25	19	31
Underweight	11	14	9
About right	63	67	58
Don't know	1	0	2

About one in six (16%) of young women claimed that they always watch what they eat because of its effect on their weight, and a further 9% of young women claimed to be currently on a restricted diet for one reason or another. Hence, a total of one in four of all young women either watch their diet closely or are on a diet, compared to only 14% of young men.

Table 4.13 Diet

	Total (502) (%)	*Men (249)* (%)	*Women (253)* (%)
I always watch what I eat because I tend to put on/lose weight easily	13	9	16
I am currently on a restricted diet to gain/lose weight	4	2	6
I am on a restricted diet for medical reasons other than weight problems	2	1	2
I am on a restricted diet for personal reasons other than weight problems	1	1	1
I am not on any restricted diet at the moment	81	87	75

Table 4.14 Importance of food

	Total (502) (%)	*Men (249)* (%)	*Women (253)* (%)
I don't think about what I eat, I eat what I like	59	68	50
I'm concerned about food because I play sport	4	6	2
I'm concerned about food because of my health	10	8	11
I'm concerned about food because of my appearance	10	6	15
I'm generally concerned about what I eat	15	9	20
None of these	3	3	3

The qualitative research revealed that young men were much less concerned about what they eat than young women and this is revealed in Table 4.14, which shows that 68% of young men compared to only 50% of young women claim to 'eat what they like'.

Amongst the remainder, concern was expressed about their food consumption because of its effect on their appearance, health or the sport they play.

For both sexes, exercise was important, with 28% claiming to exercise at least once a day. 70% of young men claimed to exercise at least once a week and similarly for women — 65% at least once a week (Table 4.15).

The study investigated the effect of smoking on appetite since the

Table 4.15 Exercise taken

	Total (502) (%)	*Men* (249) (%)	*Women* (253) (%)
Daily	28	31	26
2–3 times a week	25	28	23
Once a week	14	11	16
Less than once a week but more than once a month	5	6	4
Once a month or less	7	8	6
Never	21	16	25

Table 4.16 Affect of smoking on eating habits

	Total	*Men*	*Women*
Base — all smokers	173 (%)	87 (%)	86 (%)
None, no difference	63	69	57
Curbs nunger, dulls the appetite	14	13	16
Makes me eat less	18	15	22
Alters/spoils the taste of food	5	5	6
Other	2	1	3
Don't know	1	1	1

qualitative research revealed that some teenagers justify smoking because it helps to restrict their diet and keep their weight down.

Amongst smokers, 63% thought that smoking had no effect on their diet but amongst the remainder 22% thought it dulled their appetite or made them eat less, and a further 5% thought it spoiled the taste of food (Table 4.16).

SOURCES OF INFORMATION ABOUT DIET AND FOOD

Sources of information about diet and food varied considerably between the sexes (Table 4.17). For men, television (40%) and parents (35%) were the most important, whereas young women were much more influenced by 'other' magazines (50%), which consisted primarily of women's magazines, and friends (43%). The qualitative research revealed that many young men were taught how to cook a basic meal by their mother before they left home and their mother's advice was an important factor on their choice of food. For young women, magazines played an important role in their sources of information about diet and food and also very influencial was 'word of mouth' advice from friends.

Table 4.17 Sources of information about diet and food

	Total (*502*) (%)	*Men* (*249*) (%)	*Women* (*253*) (%)
Television	36	40	32
Radio	9	9	9
Newspapers	21	20	21
Specialist magazines	12	4	19
Other magazines	29	8	50
School/college	12	7	17
Friends	34	26	43
Parents	33	35	32
Books/cookery books	2	2	3
Other	3	2	4
Don't know	19	27	10

Approximately half of all young people (49%) claim to read food labels either often or sometimes, with the incidence of reading much higher amongst young women (57%) than young men (40%) (Table 4.18).

Table 4.18 Frequency of reading food labels

	Total *(502)* (%)	*Men* *(249)* (%)	*Women* *(253)* (%)
Often	23	18	27
Sometimes	26	22	30
Rarely	21	20	22
Never	30	40	21

Table 4.19 Concern about ingredients

	Total	*Men*	*Women*
Base—reading all labels	350 (%)	149 (%)	201 (%)
Very worried	3	2	3
Quite worried	15	7	20
Not very worried	33	33	33
Not at all worried	48	54	44
Don't know	1	3	0
Worrying ingredients			
Base—all worried	60	14	46
Colouring	48	36	52
Additives (unspecified)	42	29	46
Preservatives	37	36	37
Other	35	50	30
Emulsifiers	28	29	28
Artificial sweeteners	23	14	26
Flavouring	23	21	24
Antioxidants	18	14	20
Stablisers	18	14	20
Sugar	15	0	20
Don't know	8	14	7

Almost a quarter (23%) of young women claimed that they were quite or very worried about ingredients but only 9% of men were concerned (Table 4.19).

Table 4.20 Availability of information about ingredients

	Total (502) (%)	*Men (249)* (%)	*Women (253)* (%)
More	49	43	54
About the same	32	35	28
Less	1	1	1
Don't know	18	20	16
Where information should be provided			
Base—all saying more	245	108	137
On food labels	69	67	72
From manufacturer's leaflets	14	9	18
From the media	15	19	12
From the Government	9	12	7
Other	3	4	3
Don't know	3	4	3

Table 4.21 Perception about the term 'additives'

	Total (502) (%)	*Men (249)* (%)	*Women (253)* (%)
Colouring	31	33	30
Preservatives	25	24	26
Flavouring	22	22	22
Extras added to food	11	10	12
Spices/minerals/salts	6	7	5
Sugar/sweeteners	6	6	6
Other	5	6	5
Chemicals	4	4	4
Emulsifiers	3	2	4
Antioxidants	2	1	2
Stabilisers	2	1	4
Don't know	30	28	32

Ingredients which caused the greatest concern (amongst those who were worried and read food labels) were colouring (48%), additives (42%), preservatives (37%), emulsifiers (28%), artificial sweeteners (23%) and flavouring (23%).

Table 4.22 Daily consumption of eating food items

	Total *(504)* (%)	*Men* *(249)* (%)	*Women* *(253)* (%)
Chocolate, sugar confectionery	32	31	33
Ice-cream, lollies	1	2	0
Snack foods	29	32	26
Cooked lunch	33	40	27
Tinned vegetables	8	10	5
Tinned soup	3	4	3
Cooked evening meal	78	82	75
Dessert mixes	3	4	2

Table 4.23 Average daily food consumption

	Total *(502)* (g)	*Men* *(249)* (g)	*Women* *(253)* (g)
Chocolates and other sweets	25	30	20
Crisps, nuts, etc.	15	15	15
Soft drinks	185	185	185
Milk as a drink	105	130	75
Alcoholic drinks	245	395	100
Meat and fish	135	155	110
Eggs and cheese	45	50	45
Vegetables	200	230	175
Fruit	55	55	60
Puddings and cakes	55	60	55
Bread	110	135	85
Biscuits	15	15	15
Breakfast cereals	10	15	10

(From Bull, 1985)

Half of all respondents wanted more information about constituents of food and most of these wanted to see the information on the food labels themselves (69%). Only a small proportion wanted manufacturers' leaflets (14%) and a sizeable proportion of men would like more information to be provided by the media (19%) (Table 4.20).

In summary, there is considerable interest, and in some cases concern, about food ingredients and manufacturers should provide details of food constituents on the labels.

Respondents were questioned about their concept of additives and the responses are shown in Table 4.21. Colouring heads the list (31%), followed by preservatives (25%) and flavouring (22%).

Table 4.24 Foods one likes but feels one shouldn't eat

	Total (502) (%)	*Men (249)* (%)	*Women (253)* (%)
Chips	17	14	19
Crisps	5	2	8
Potatoes	1	1	2
Fried fatty foods	6	7	5
Cakes/buns	9	6	13
Cream cakes	4	1	7
Puddings	1	1	1
Pastry	1	1	0
Bread	2	1	4
Cheese	3	2	4
Other dairy products	4	4	4
Meat	2	2	1
Meat products	3	4	3
Chocolate	19	11	27
Sweets/toffees	11	7	14
Sugar	1	1	1
Other sweet foods	3	2	4
Soft/fizzy drinks	1	0	1
Pasta	2	0	3
Other	6	5	7
Don't know	37	51	23

Emulsifiers and antioxidants were recalled by only 2 or 3% of young people.

Table 4.22 gives details of claimed daily consumption of certain food items. Almost four out of five respondents claimed to have a cooked evening meal but one in three claimed to have a cooked lunch — rising to 40% amongst men, but only 27% amongst women. Men have more cooked lunches than women because of the lunches provided at work or they visit a cafe or a pub.

Table 4.23 gives details of the average daily food consumption in grams as estimated from the diary exercise.

Table 4.24 reveals that chocolates, chips, sweets and toffees are the foods which young people like but feel that they shouldn't eat. In spite of this, one in three eat chocolate and sugar confectionery daily!

Table 4.25 reveals that 'eat your greens' is still the phrase ringing in young people's ears, because greens and other vegetables,

Table 4.25 Disliked foods which one feels one ought to eat

	Total *(502)* (%)	*Men* *(249)* (%)	*Women* *(253)* (%)
Cabbage	6	7	5
Greens/green vegetables	12	12	11
Other vegetables	16	16	15
Salad/salad vegetables	4	4	3
Fruit	2	2	2
Liver	16	8	24
Other offal	3	3	3
Meat	4	3	6
Fish	6	4	9
Cheese	3	2	4
Eggs	2	3	2
Milk	2	1	4
Bran/bran food	1	1	1
Other	4	3	6
Don't know	41	46	36

together with liver, are the most disliked foods which they feel they ought to eat.

Lastly, one in 20 young people claim a food allergy but this is much higher amongst women (8%) than men (2%).

Table 4.26 Food allergies

	Total (502) (%)	*Men (249)* (%)	*Women (253)* (%)
Yes	5	2	8
No	95	98	92

References

Bull, N. L. (1985). Dietary habits of 15 to 25-year-olds. *Hum. Nutr. Appl. Nutr.*, **39A**, Suppl. 1

Gallup (1974–1985). The British Survey of Eating Out.

Gallup (1984/1985). Menu and Business Survey. *Caterer and Hotelkeeper, 1984, 1985.*

5
Fast foods

J. M. PASCOE, J. DOCKERTY AND J. RYLEY

ABSTRACT

Studies on the nutrient content of fast and take-away foods have been reported from the United States and Australia, but data in the UK have been sparse. Recently, some of the fast food chains have published their own data.

A study currently being carried out at Leeds University, and financed by MAFF, has included fast foods, fish and chips, other traditional products and a range of ethnic foods.

In recent months in the UK, nutritional concerns have focused on the findings of the Committee on the Medical Aspects of Food Policy, COMA (1984). Some of the results of the Leeds study will be presented and discussed in the context of the recommendations of this report. However, it is important to remember that the recommendations refer to the whole diet and can be misleading if applied to single meals or menu items.

INTRODUCTION

Fast food is best defined not as a product, but as a system of technology which can be applied to many different foods and situations. The term describes the American system of food service, represented by the modern counter service units of Burger King, Wimpy and McDonald, and also other styles of restaurant including some pizza and chicken outlets and fish and chip shops.

'Take-away' food is a wider term which may refer to fast food, but may also encompass almost any type of meal or snack if it has been prepared, probably hot, and individually packaged for immediate consumption off the premises.

In financial terms, in 1984, ethnic take-aways (£215 million) and fish and chip shops (£470 million) combined had a market share approximately equal to that of the fast food chains' take-away outlets (£670 million) (*Popular Food Service*, 1984). The projected sales for 1990 show a 250% sales increase for the fast food chains, with ethnic outlets and fish and chip shops static. Sales of fast food comprise 69% from burger outlets, 12% from pizza outlets and 14% from chicken outlets. Chinese take-aways have the largest proportion of the turnover of the ethnic take-aways (60%).

There is a need for composition data on the products of the catering industry as a whole, of which take-aways constitute 25% of meal occasions (Heald, ibid). Detailed analytical studies on the nutrient content of fast and take-away foods have been carried out in the US by Appledorf (1974) and by the fast food chains (*FDA Consumer*, 1983), and have been summarised by Khan and Rao (1983). A wide range of Australian items has been analysed by Greenfield and Wills *et al.*, and reported in a series of papers (Wills and Greenfield, 1980; Wills *et al.*, 1981a; Greenfield *et al.*, 1981; Wills and Greenfield, 1981; Wills *et al.*, 1981b; Greenfield *et al.*, 1982). However, there are no such reports from the UK, although recently the fast food chains have been publishing their own data (McDonald's Hamburgers Ltd., 1985; Wimpy International Ltd., 1985). Popular magazines such as *Which?* (1985) and *Slimming Magazine* (1984) have compiled useful lists, as has *Balance* (Metcalfe and Hall, 1984), the instrument of the British Diabetic Association.

An analytical study of the composition of 150 fast and take-away menu items in London and the North of England has been undertaken by Pascoe, Dockerty and Ryley with a grant from the Ministry of Agriculture, Fisheries and Food. The details of this study, which includes macronutrients, water- and fat-soluble vitamins and some minerals, will be reported in appropriate journals. The aspects discussed in this chapter are protein, carbohydrate and fat content, energy, proportion of energy from fat, polyunsaturated to saturated fatty acid ratio (P:S) and sodium content, and include some of the issues on which UK dietary concerns have been focused in recent months.

SELECTION OF TYPES OF TAKE-AWAY AND FOOD

The outlets from which samples were collected reflected their importance in market surveys of turnover and included fish and chip shops, burger, chicken and pizza bars, Chinese, Indian, Greek and Italian take-aways, baked potato outlets and outlets selling 'traditional' items such as pork pies and sausage rolls.

There are regional differences in the types of fast/take-away outlets. For example, American-type burger establishments are more common in the South than in the North of England. Methods of preparation and cooking may also vary regionally, as do patterns of consumption. Therefore, food samples were collected in London and in the North of England. Most of the samples from the North were collected in Leeds but some sampling in Manchester, Sheffield and York was undertaken because the range was too limited in Leeds.

It was not possible within the scope of this study to collect every menu item from each type of take-away. A sample of between four and seven foods, which were judged to be representative of the menus, was selected from each variety of take-away.

Collection and preparation of samples

Once the range of food samples for the particular outlet type had been selected, six premises serving these items were found in the area. The foods were then purchased hot from each outlet as if by a consumer, cooled in solid carbon dioxide and returned to the laboratory, where the individual portions were weighed. The six portions were then homogenised together to obtain a composite sample for analysis. Labile nutrients were analysed immediately and the remaining sample stored at −20 °C until required for analysis.

Regional differences

Figure 5.1 illustrates typical compositional differences found between similar products collected in Leeds and London. In general, portions from fish and chip shops and ethnic restaurants were larger in London and contained more fat, protein and carbohydrate and total energy than Leeds meals. The polyunsaturated to saturated (P:S) fatty acid ratio was lower in Leeds, indicating a greater use of saturated fat. However, the composition of the products of individual chains and the fatty acid composition of the fat were similar in both Leeds and London.

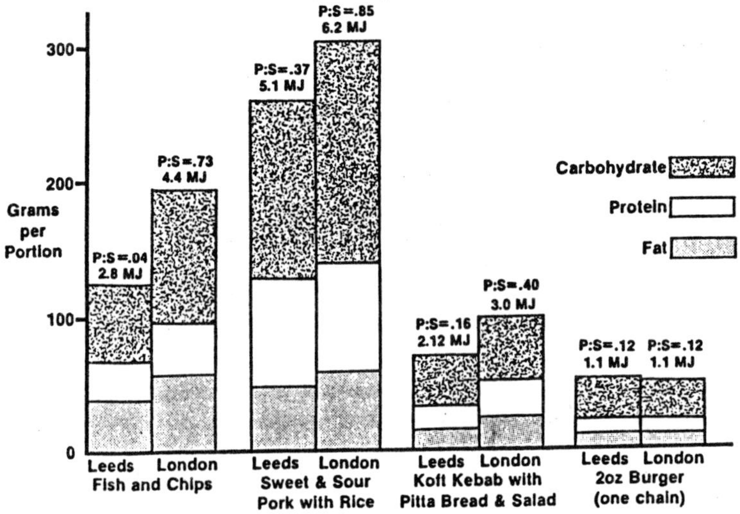

Figure 5.1 Comparison of meals from Leeds and London

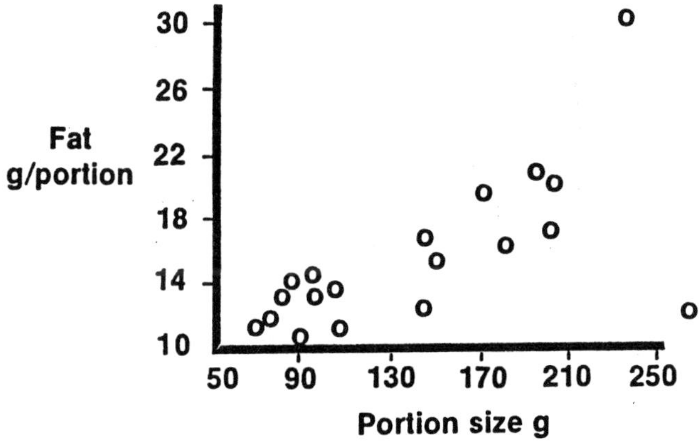

Figure 5.2 Chips—relationship between fat per portion and portion size

Chips

Chips are served with one meal in three in the catering industry and probably constitute the most important single menu item. Portions from small shops had a mean energy value of 1.79 ± 0.66* MJ and those from the chains 1.10 ± 0.08 MJ per portion, but both the fat content and the portion size were very variable.

Figure 5.2 shows the relationship between fat content and portion size for standard portions collected from chains and small operators in London and the North of England. The smaller portions came from the fast food chains and the larger from the fish and chip shops. In general, larger portions contained more fat per portion than small portions, as would be expected. The mean value for the products of chain operators was 12.0 ± 0.83 grams fat per portion and is similar to values reported from the US (Khan and Rao, 1983). The mean portion size was 129 ± 14 grams in Leeds and 119 ± 6 grams in London. For chips from small operators, the mean fat content was 20.4 ± 4.8 grams per portion, with an average portion size of 194 ± 9 grams in Leeds and 230 ± 33 grams in London.

* All figures are mean ± standard error of mean (SEM). 1 MJ = 239 kcal

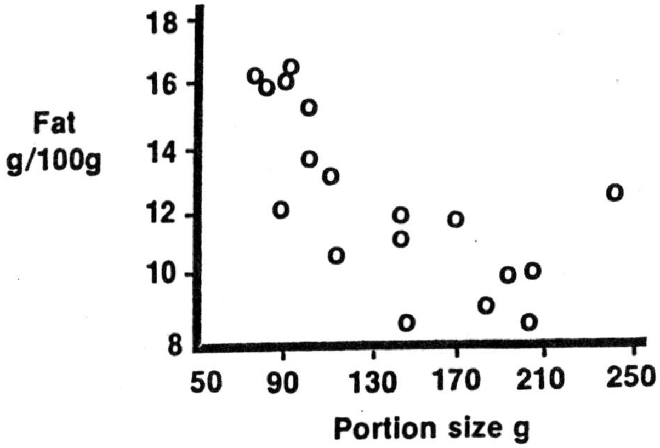

Figure 5.3 'French fries' — relationship between composition and portion size

A thin product popularly described as 'French fries' and associated with some chains presents a greater surface for fat absorption and moisture loss than 'chips', which have a larger cross-sectional area. Figure 5.3 shows that a higher percentage fat was associated with the products sold in small portions. Small portions were mainly from chains and in the form normally called 'French fries'.

A laboratory study (Greenfield *et al.*, 1984) has shown that the common domestic procedure of one-stage frying gives a final fat content in the range of 4–12 grams per 100 grams, whereas the industrial process of two-stage frying gives 8–19 grams per 100 grams. Figure 5.3 shows that the range of values for products collected in Leeds and London had a fat content in the range of 8–17 grams per 100 grams. This is very similar to the range reported by Greenfield *et al.* for Australian products, who concluded that their results were characteristic of two-stage frying (Greenfield *et al.*, 1984).

The fatty acid composition of the fried potato products studied by Pascoe *et al.* ranged from polyunsaturated to saturated fatty acid (P:S) of 0.051:1 for chips in Leeds to 0.74:1 for chips in London, with products from chains in the range 0.1:1 to 0.38:1. These results indicate considerable use of saturated fats in fish and chip shops in Leeds and amongst the chains, but fish and chip shops in London seemed to be using oils with a high content of polyunsaturates.

Macronutrient content

Table 5.1 and Figure 5.4 compare different aspects of the composition of typical items purchased in Leeds from each type of outlet examined.

Traditional bakery items such as pork pies, steak pies, Cornish pasties and sausage rolls are sold in small portions in the range 1–2 MJ. The proportion of fat in this group of products (48–57% of energy) was amongst the highest encountered and substantially higher than either the current average UK diet (42% energy from fat) or the COMA recommended level of 35% (DHSS, 1984). However, they all contributed more than 10% of the recommended daily amount (RDA) of protein for both men and women. A content of 10% RDA is the lowest level generally utilised to identify a useful dietary source. The P:S ratio, although lower than in the

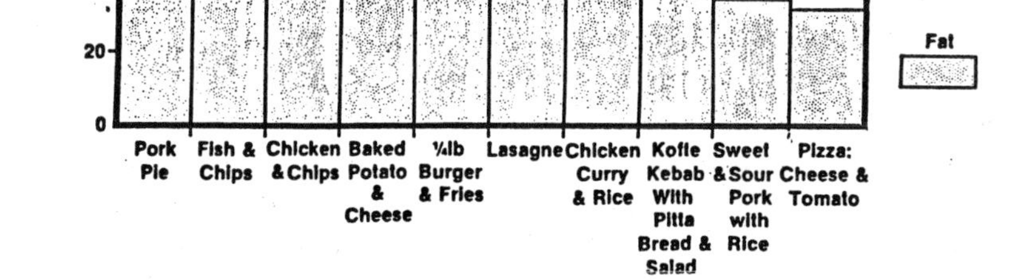

Figure 5.4 Breakdown of energy contribution — Leeds samples

majority of products analysed, nevertheless exceeded the COMA recommended minimum of 0.23 (DHSS, 1984).

Fish and chips from small shops in Leeds contained, on average, 2.8 MJ of energy — less than one-third RDA for both men and women. The fat content of 38.7 grams was approximately equally divided between the chips and the batter, and contributed 51% of the total energy of the meal. Fish and chips is a major source of protein, contributing 34% RDA for men and 46% for women.

Chicken and chips from a chain operator had a very similar protein content to fish and chips, but less fat and therefore less total energy. Nevertheless, the proportion of energy from fat was high (46.9%).

Baked potatoes constitute a new type of take-away item with a 'healthy' image. The fat content ranged from 10.9 grams per portion when buttered to 26 grams (a surprising 45% energy from fat) when filled with cheese. Baked potatoes with cheese have a similar fat and protein content to chicken and chips but 16% more carbohydrate.

Pizzas. 'Thin pizzas' from chains fell in the range 2.6–3.3 MJ per portion and 'deep pan pizzas' in the range 3.1–3.7 MJ per portion. Thus, the cheese and tomato pizza depicted in Table 5.1 and Figure 5.4 for a mixed sample collected in Leeds is larger than average (4 MJ). The percentage energy from fat for pizzas was often below 35% and rarely exceeded 40%. The P:S ratio was variable but tended to be low since many pizzas incorporated substantial amounts of cheese. Pizzas are massive contributors to protein intake. The Leeds sample quoted in Table 5.1 contains 92% of RDA of protein for women.

Burgers. The term 'burger' includes the bun, the filling and the dressing. The most popular sales combination is the ¼ lb burger served with fries. The Leeds example contained 3.1 MJ of energy and 36 grams of fat of which nearly two-thirds is in the burger and constitutes 43% of the total energy of the combination. The protein content was substantial (57% RDA for women). The more exotic burgers with cheese or larger quantities of meat and dressing and served with fries contained up to 45 grams of fat and the proportion of energy from fat of the combination exceeded 50%. A standard

Table 5.1 Composition of fast/take-away meals in Leeds (per portion)

Item	*Portion size* (g)	*Fat* (g)	*Protein* (g)	*Total CHO*[a] (g)	*Total energy* (MJ)	*% recommended daily amount* *Protein*		*Energy*	
						M	*W*	*M*	*W*
Pork pie	123	26.3	12.5	31.9	1.7	17.4	23.1	14.2	18.9
Fish and chips	299	38.7	24.7	60.6	2.8	34.3	45.7	23.3	31.1
Chicken and chips (no bone)	220	26.6	22.5	44.8	2.1	31.3	41.7	17.5	23.3
Baked potato with cheese	298	26.0	20.4	52.1	2.1	28.3	37.8	17.5	23.3
¼ lb burger with fries	315	35.9	30.8	81.7	3.1	42.8	57.0	25.8	34.4
Lasagne	538	33.4	40.0	63.3	2.9	32.2	43.0	24.2	32.2
Sweet and sour pork with rice	597	48.2	30.5	180.2	5.2	42.4	56.5	43.3	57.8
Chicken curry with rice	615	37.8	39.4	94.5	3.6	54.7	73.0	30.0	40.0
Kofte kebab with pitta bread and salad	220	14.5	17.8	40.7	1.5	24.7	33.0	12.5	16.7
Pizza (cheese and tomato)	351	33.4	49.9	111.5	4.0	69.3	92.4	33.3	44.4
RDA (18–35-year-old man moderately active)			72		12				
RDA (18–54-year-old woman)			54		9				

[a] expressed as monosaccharide

2 oz burger with fries contained only 22 grams of fat and 41% energy from fat.

Products from ethnic outlets. Table 5.1 and Figure 5.4 include typical examples of Chinese, Indian, Italian and Greek take-away foods. Often entrée items incorporated a substantial quantity of a staple starchy food (e.g., pasta dishes, kebabs in pitta bread and sweet and sour pork with rice) so that the percentage energy from fat tended to be moderate, at 40% or less. The range of energy values was very wide, with Indian meals being, in general, the largest, and Greek the smallest. Sweet and sour pork was exceptionally high (5.1 MJ in Leeds), probably due to the large sugar content (approximately 50 grams per portion). As the ethnic entrées tended to be large, they contained significant quantities of fat and protein. Sweet and sour pork with rice contained more fat (48 grams) than any other combination of entrée and staple studied, except battered plaice with chips purchased in London, which contained 60 grams of fat. The P:S ratio of the fat in ethnic products was very variable, ranging from 0.07:1 for kebabs, which contain only the fat remaining in the meat, to 1.85:1 for a vegetable curry collected in London, and reflects the wide range of ingredients and cooking processes.

Sodium

Table 5.2 shows the mean sodium content of products collected from Leeds and London. Values range from 0.14 ± 0.11 to 1.68 ± 0.63 grams of sodium per portion. When expressed per unit of energy, the results fall in the range 0.15 ± 0.03 to 0.72 ± 0.04 grams of sodium per MJ.

Estimates of the mean sodium intake per day in the UK have yielded values of between 2.7 and 4.0 grams per day (without discretionary salt addition) (BNF, 1985a). Thus a hypothetical person eating fast/take-away foods for total energy requirements (10 MJ/day for men and 8 MJ for women) would be likely to exceed this figure, particularly if their choice included ethnic foods or bacon products.

Table 5.2 Sodium content of fast/take-away foods

Item	*Sodium* (g/portion)	*Sodium* (g/MJ)
Italian	1.68 ± 0.63	0.64 ± 0.19
Chinese	1.58 ± 0.50	0.67 ± 0.26
Pizzas	1.41 ± 0.20	0.44 ± 0.05
Greek	1.08 ± 0.35	0.57 ± 0.08
Indian	1.04 ± 0.40	0.57 ± 0.18
Chicken/bun	0.97 ± 0.20	0.49 ± 0.07
Bacon/bun	0.93 ± 0.25	0.72 ± 0.04
'Superburgers'	0.90 ± 0.59	0.43 ± 0.07
Pastry products (savoury)	0.71 ± 0.22	0.43 ± 0.06
Cheeseburgers (2 oz)	0.70 ± 0.15	0.53 ± 0.53
Basic burgers (chain, 2 oz)	0.52 ± 0.07	0.48 ± 0.11
Baked potatoes (3 kinds)	0.45 ± 0.31	0.24 ±0.06
Fried fish	0.40 ± 0.18	0.24 ± 0.14
Fried chicken	0.40 ± 0.10	0.50 ± 0.12
Desserts	0.21 ± 0.14	0.16 ± 0.04
Fries/chips	0.14 ± 0.11	0.15 ± 0.03

Mean ± 2 SEM

CONCLUSION

Although the major consumers of fast and take-away foods are known to be 16–25-year-olds (Gallup, 1980, 1981; BNF, 1985b), the estimate of their contribution to the total diet is very small. In a recent study of the dietary habits of 15–25-year-olds (Bull, 1985) the average number of restaurant and take-away meals per person was only 0.77 per 14-day period. On this basis, it may be concluded that the composition of meals in this area is a matter of interest rather than a matter of importance, except for the convenience of people with special dietary requirements, such as diabetics.

Nevertheless, it should be remembered that averages mask extremes. The type of product favoured by this sector of the catering industry is often high in fat (fish and chips, traditional bakery items) or high in sodium (Chinese meals) or both.

However, many of them constitute major protein sources and are often high in polyunsaturates. Some sectors of the market produce products with a very low P:S ratio, notably fish and chip shops in Leeds and chips from the fast food chains. It seems likely that consumer pressures will promote increased use of unsaturated oils for frying operations.

References

Appledorf, H. (1984). Nutritional analysis of foods from fast food chains. *Food Technol.*, April, 51–5

British Nutrition Foundation (1985a). *Salt in the Diet*, Briefing Paper No. 7

British Nutrition Foundation (1985b). *Eating in the Early 1980s Attitudes and Behaviour — Main Findings*

Bull, N. L. (1985). Dietary habits of 15 to 25-year-olds. *Hum. Nutr. Appl. Nutr.*, **39A**, Suppl. 1, 1–68

Department of Health and Social Security (1984). *Diet and Cardio-vascular Disease*. Report on Health and Social Subjects, No. 28. (HMSO, London)

FDA Consumer (1983). 'A Look at Fast Food Nutrients', pp 14–15

Gallup (1980 and 1981). *British Survey of Eating Out*

Greenfield, H., Wimalasiri, P., Han, L. T. N., Balmer, N. and Wills, R. B. H. (1981). Composition of Australian foods 6. Chinese foods. *Food Technol. Aust.*, **33** (4), 176–81

Greenfield, H., Wimalasiri, P., Ma, S. N. N. and Wills, R. B. H. (1982). Composition of Australian foods 16. Food from Pizza Hut Restaurants. *Food Technol. Aust.*, **34** (8), 364–7

Greenfield, H., Makinson, J. and Wills, R. B. H. (1984). Lipids in French fries: a retail and laboratory study. *J. Food Technol.*, **19**, 239–45

Heald, G. Ibid.

Khan, M. A. and Rao, R. M. (1983). Nutritional quality of meals served by selected foodservices. *CRC Crit. Rev. Food Sci. Nutr.*, **19** (2), 151–71

McDonald's Hamburgers Ltd. (1985). *Nutritional Analysis of Foods served at McDonald's Restaurants*. (Public Relations Dept., McDonald's Hamburgers Ltd.)

Metcalfe, J. and Hall, S. (1984). 'Have diabetes, will travel and eat — no trouble'. *Balance*, June, 12–13

Popular Food Service, October 1984

Slimming Magazine (1984). 'Your greatest guide to calories'

Which?, February 1985, 54–7

Wills, R. B. H. and Greenfield, H. (1980). Composition of Australian foods 3. Foods from a major fast food chain. *Food Technol. Aust.*, **32**, 363–6

Wills, R. B. H. and Greenfield, H. (1981). Composition of Australian foods 8. Fortification of McDonald's foods. *Food Technol. Aust.*, **33** (8), 378–80

Wills, R. B. H., Wimalasiri, P. and Greenfield, H. (1981a). Composition of Australian foods 5. Fried take-away foods. *Food Technol. Aust.*, **33** (1), 26–7

Wills, R. B. H., Makinson, J. and Greenfield, H. (1981b). Composition of Australian foods 9. Meat pies, sausage rolls and pasties. *Food Technol. Aust.*, **33** (9), 450–4

Wimpy Fact Sheet 1 (1985). *Fast Food and Healthy Eating*. (Wimpy International Ltd.)

6
The impact of nutritional and health concepts on catering practice within the school meals service

T. A. BALL

ABSTRACT

The origins of the school meals service were founded on the nutritional needs of less privileged children. During both World Wars the nutritional intake of children taking school meals was enhanced over and above that of the general public. The Education Act 1944 provided for the setting up of the modern school meals service with simple nutritional guidelines linked to a recommended pattern of food buying. By 1975 over 70% of pupils were taking school meals but the percentage has now dropped to 51.3%.

The section of the Education Act 1980 that dealt with meals was conceived against a financial decision to seek a 50% reduction in the net expenditure on school meals. Central nutritional guidelines were dropped and a statutory duty was imposed to allow pupils to bring their own sandwich meals. The emphasis, particularly in secondary schools, switched from a fixed charge meal, usually with choice, to a multi-choice cash cafeteria and the imposed commercial approach made it almost impossible to guide the customer towards a healthy diet.

A wind of change, possibly only a zephyr at present, has now been detected. Co-operation is at last being established among caterers, home economists and dietitians, linked to a greater awareness on the part of the general public. This movement is resulting in the production, marketing and, most importantly, consumption of 'better' foodstuffs in terms of the current nutritional recommendations.

DISCUSSION

The origins of the school meals service were founded on the nutritional needs of the less privileged children in our society and the service can be traced back to the work of various charities in the mid-19th century. The first Government involvement came with the Education (Provision of Meals) Act 1906 that allowed Local Education Authorities to take such steps as they thought fit for the provision of meals at any public elementary school. Then, during both World Wars, considerable attention was paid to ensuring school children received a reasonably nutritious diet in times of general hardship as far as national food supplies were concerned.

The modern service was finally established within the Education Act 1944 and delineated by subsequent regulations. The principles then applied were succinctly spelled out in Circular 97 of 1946:–

> 'The school dinner is one of the most important and frequent occasions on which large numbers of the pupils are assembled together to act as a community ... under proper conditions it affords an outstanding opportunity for social training, without which education is incomplete, for teaching good manners and for the establishment of sound dietetic habits.'

From those sturdy seeds sown in 1944 the service continued to grow until by the late 1960s and early 1970s over 5 million pupils were taking a school meal each day; at the peak this represented over 70% of all pupils present. At that time, meals were provided to simple nutritional guidelines aimed at attaining target nutritional levels of 29 g protein, 32 g fat and 880 kcals. One criticism, among many of that system, was that the guidance was based on food as purchased rather than on food on the plate. The Department attempted to monitor the nutritional value of food purchased by kitchen returns from a selection of schools using nutritional tables. The typical meal then was produced within a standard menu system sometimes offering a simple choice of two dishes, but any information the Department received on nutrition may well have been accompanied by substantial figures for waste both in the preparation of the meal and from the plate — resulting in a dilution of the nutritional intake. So, to some extent, the old service took refuge in paper nutritional figures.

In 1973 a detailed review of school catering took place, with two associated reports published in 1975. There was much good sense in both these reports and I would like to quote just one paragraph from each:–

> *Catering in Schools*
> '19. It should be the service's general aim to provide main meals and other refreshment which are not only attractive to the pupils but also make good sense in terms of their nutritional needs. By this we mean, in the case of a main mid-day meal, one which makes at least the contribution to a child's nutritional needs that he would expect to get from a good sustaining meal at home, and which also contributes to his longer-term growth needs. We know that there are difficulties. A meal that nutritionists would regard as well-nourishing and balanced may not be attractive to pupils. A set mid-day meal at school may not fit in with a family's routine for the day. What pupils, especially some older pupils, want to eat at mid-day would not, when considered in isolation, always be regarded with approbation by nutritionists. Some balance must be struck between nutritional aims and the taste of the consumer. There is no merit in a well-balanced and nourishing meal which remains uneaten.'

> *Nutrition in Schools — Introduction*
> '3. On more than one occasion we have found ourselves discussing the school meal in the broader context of education, the fostering of good eating habits in younger children and the encouragement of intelligent interest in the choice and preparation of food in older pupils. While the emphasis throughout this report has necessarily been on the nutritional aspects of catering, we would not want it to be thought that eating has been seen merely as "refuelling", to the neglect of what is creative and imaginative in the choice, preparation and presentation of food. We welcome the moves that are being made to bring the school catering service into closer working relationship with home economics departments in schools. We commend curricular links of this nature as a promising way of creating an awareness of healthy eating habits as an enjoyable and satisfying aspect of the art of living.'

Excellent though these two reports may have been — as has been apparent in so many similar situations — the time was not right. The Government of the day was already beginning to put pressure on the school meals service.

In addition to the official Department reports on school meals, there have been a number of other studies and reports commenting *inter alia* on the nutritional aspects of the service. To mention just two, Professor Bender drew attention to some of the failings in a London Borough and one of the home counties, and in 1981 the National Dairy Council in conjunction with the BNF reported on the eating habits of school children. Regrettably, there have also been reports, often popular magazine based, that have attempted to sensationalise the situation and in many cases the methodology of such surveys has been extremely suspect. At the time of writing we still await the results of the DHSS survey on school meals but the report by Surrey University on the school meals service in Inner London Education Authority Secondary Schools produced some useful data on the eating habits of school children and some excellent recommendations concerning nutrition education.

By the late 1970s successive Governments were increasingly concerned at the level of financial subsidy carried by school catering — though in fairness to the caterers, blame for the level of subsidy in the main lay fairly on these self-same Governments. With the Education Act 1980 the present Government dropped national nutritional guidelines for school meals and left it to each individual authority to set its own meal standards for pupils qualifying for free meals, or to use the wording of Section 22 of the Act: 'to ensure that such provision is made for him (the free meal pupil) in the middle of the day as appears to the authority to be requisite'. You will note a remarkable similarity with the wording of the 1906 Act. The dropping of nutritional guidelines was subsequently challenged by a Select Committee of the Commons. In the 7th Report from the Education, Science and Arts Committee in 1982, their first recommendation called on the Department to determine new nutritional standards with the authority to impose a minimum standard if Local Education Authorities ignored such advice on nutrition. The Government's response was to reject this recommendation.

What we then had was a varying picture developing across the country. In many cases, but not all, the response by individual Local Education Authorities to the freedom granted in Section 22 of the Act was conditioned by the colour of the ruling political party. The majority of the Authorities have sought to introduce a choice of menu in order to combat waste and this choice can range from a simple two-choice, two-course menu through to a multi-choice either for a set charge or on a cash basis — the so-called cash cafeteria. Generally speaking, the greater the degree of choice, the less the control that can be exercised over nutritional intake. In association with this widening of choice there also developed a much more commercial approach to the meal service. It could truly be said that the school meals service changed almost overnight from a social service to a quasi-commercial catering operation.

I apologise for spending so long on the preamble to this chapter but it is important to set the scene and clarify the situation. If I had been asked the question as recently as twelve months ago, 'What is the impact of nutrition and health concepts on school catering policy?', I am sure I would have answered with a definite 'There is no impact!'. However, much to my own surprise, the situation has already begun to change and the speed of change appears to be constantly accelerating.

I really estimate the impact of all the varying reports on nutrition — at least on the general public and, within this I include school children — as pretty low but there is no doubt in my mind that the two *World in Action* programmes on TV suddenly jolted everyone out of a state of complacency. The caterer, of course, is still faced with the same problem — at least in most Local Authorities. He or she can only survive by providing what the customer will eat and pay for!

Against this commercial background let me now explain what has been happening in the field. First we saw the development of individual action by the caterers. Examples of such action would be the setting up of salad bars; in one Authority even extending to self-help salad bars for infant school children. In these there would usually be a plated protein element, e.g., quiche, and the children would then help themselves to the various salads, guided by a member of the kitchen staff or a supervisory assistant; many Authorities had been using a mixture of wholemeal and white flour for some time but such items were now given more prominence on the menu. In general, it has been found that school children do not like 100% wholemeal flour items but will select and enjoy items using a mixed flour. Then there was the selective pricing approach, also reflected in the so-called star choice fixed price system — here items that the caterer felt could be detrimental if purchased to excess, e.g., chips, were proportionately more expensive to purchase than, say, baked jacket potatoes.

The latest development, and note I use the word 'latest' rather than 'final', is the one that I really see as a great source of encouragement. This has been, at long last, a coming together of the various factions involved — home economics teachers and advisers, community dietitians and the caterers.

An immediate problem, of course, is — what does one mean by good nutritional advice? I found considerable comfort in the commonsense advice given by Professor Macdonald at last year's BNF Annual Lecture: 'Nutrition in Balance — Fact and Fantasy'. Caterers as a breed tend to have both feet firmly on the ground, unlike some of their more scientific colleagues, so they will always err on the side of a cautious approach to the problem. They will readily take the current recommendations to heart — more fibre, less fat, sugar and salt — but draw the line at excess, at least in terms of nutritional advice.

Examples of the incidence of nutritional co-operation are far too numerous now for me to do anything but quote a few specific cases I have come across. In Leicestershire we have a community dietitian working closely to develop 'Healthy Eating Fortnights'. An interesting observation reported from one of these experiments was that when the full range of potato varieties was available on a servery counter, jacket potatoes outsold chips by a ratio of five to one. Norfolk has introduced Health Food Trolleys, Health Bars, and Health Snack Packs, and has reintroduced a star choice system in junior school cafeterias to try to guide pupils in a wiser choice. Cambridgeshire advises parents and pupils that its kitchens now use only polyunsaturated fats. Somerset is detailing relative energy, fat, sugar and fibre levels of all dishes sold by their County Catering Service. Sheffield is removing salt cellars from tables back to the servery counter and is cutting back on salt and sugar in all its recipes, but one of their kitchen supervisors summed up her problems when she said 'Meal planners are having to tread a careful path between keeping up with new thinking on health and still preparing food that is acceptable to the children.'

If I can now attempt to sum up the situation today I would say that the caterer is beginning to respond to nutritional advice probably because for the very first time he or she is now no longer acting in isolation but is being assisted by an educational approach in the classroom and in the community at large. In conclusion I would like to quote from one of the recommendations in the Surrey University Survey: 'It is particularly important that the nutrition educator should recognise the particular expertise with food which is possessed by the caterer and co-operate fully to ensure that the aim of guiding children towards a wise choice of food from the cash-cafeterias is realised.'

7
Hospitals

A. R. HORTON

ABSTRACT

Catering managers working in hospitals are aware of the special importance of appropriate nutrition in their stewardship for both patients and staff. Their awareness is constantly reinforced by the work of dietitians in the health-care team. They have to take current concepts and apply them not only to groups of people with some common basis of need but also specifically to meet the needs of individuals. Needs and wants have to be reconciled.

The first aim for health service catering is to provide meals that are safe, suitable (including nutritionally appropriate) and likely to be well regarded by the patient, the member of staff and the visitor.

The range of needs and wants is greater than in any other sector of the catering industry. Consider for example:

(1) Age — from young babies to the very old.
(2) Health states — the hearty eating young orthopaedic patient and the energetic student nurse to those recovering from major surgery.
(3) Therapeutic diets — an essential part of treatment that may include the 'exception to prove the rule'.
(4) Culture and religion — habits, prejudices and obligations; and each of those factors interacting with the others in the same catering unit.

Consider the logistic problems of catering in the different hospital locations: the old and the new buildings; the square mile campus and the high rise blocks; the hospital with less than twenty patients and those with over a thousand; the broad types of hospital — the famous 'teaching' names, the District Generals with many specialities, those for psychiatric treatment and those caring for the mentally handicapped. Provision is made for the metabolic units, the renal units, bone marrow transplant and so on, including irradiated meals. All these variations require particular consideration with adaptation of catering systems and methods to best meet the need. Similarly wide variations are to be found in the staff catering services.

The hospital caterer is not in sole command of the whole catering operation but depends heavily on the work and enthusiasm of others. Obviously, they rely on nursing, medical and domestic service staff, not so obviously, perhaps, on finance, supplies, personnel and general administration. Crucial for those who would make change and advance new concepts is the active support of recently appointed General Managers.

The effect of financial control — revenue and capital — the influence of national and local policies, including the current competitive tendering exercise and implications of the recent Rayner-type scrutiny of hospital catering, should all receive attention when we discuss the impact of nutrition and health concepts on catering practice in hospitals.

DISCUSSION

'Give me neither poverty nor riches;
Feed me with food convenient for me.'

(Proverbs 30, 8)

In the several countries and dependancies comprising Britain there are some 2860 hospitals, about 2630 in the National Health Service and about 230 maintained by charitable organisations or commercial enterprises owned by British or foreign investors. For the most part the work of hospitals continues through twenty-four hours a day every day.

Considering NHS hospitals in England, there are about 280 000 resident patients and 790 000 staff to be catered for by a catering staff of about 35 000 people.

More than half the registered dietitians in Britain work in NHS hospitals, providing nutrition and dietetic services. They have a duty to ensure that suitable food is available for all patients and in staff catering services. District dietitians also have responsibilities in the community at large. Health Education or Health Promotion Units are important persuaders and are busily promoting 'Healthy Eating'. Community Health Councils, 'watch dogs' for the consumers, i.e., the patients, turn their attention to catering services and there are many associations with general and sectional interests making their views and concerns on dietary matters felt at local and national levels.

Catering managers are responsible for the quality of the meals provided and they are appropriately trained, qualified and experienced people. Unfortunately, the status and salaries attached to some key posts have been reduced in recent years.

Nonetheless, catering management continues to endeavour to apply current thinking on nutrition in order to meet the individual needs of patients. The current average cost of meals provided in hospitals is £1.26 per day for food and £1.24 for wages. (This is the average actual cost in England in 1983/84 and is not an allowance. Each Health Authority sets its own budget.) When 'healthy eating' coincides with lower prices the cost-conscious hospital managers rejoice. I sense a greater enthusiasm for skimmed milk than I do for polyunsaturated margarine. Both are, of course, being used to cut down the saturated fats in the normal diet. In the past, similar coincidences gave rise to the 'poached fish and boiled rice pudding' image and before that the 'boiled mutton and weak ale' as typical hospital fare. Now, however, a greater variety of food is prepared to meet more closely the needs and wants of patients and staff, as they perceive them. When that perception coincides with the nutritionists' evidence of what is 'good for them', there is happiness all round. More often there has to be a compromise. Similarly, with methods of preparation and cooking there can be happy coincidence. In the past many hospital kitchens have had insufficient frying capacity and have substituted baked dishes. Now that has become a desirable feature of the menu.

The first aim for hospital catering is to provide meals that are safe, suitable (including nutritionally suitable) and likely to be well regarded by the patients, staff and other recipients.

It is reasonable to expect that this aim will not be met for everyone, everywhere, at the same time, but currently public concern with nutrition is helping. Many Authorities have declared 'Healthy Eating Policies' and many others, without a formal statement, are leading their people towards diets which conform to current nutritional advice.

The needs of individuals have to be met within that general philosophy, considering:–

(1) *Age* — patients from the newly born to those in the care of the geriatrician. The elderly are a large group. Hospital staff vary from the young energetic manual worker to the bench-bound ageing technologist and those in sedentary clerical and administative jobs.

(2) *State of health* — from the convalescent orthopaedic patient to the obese or the undernourished awaiting or recovering from major surgery. From the hospital football team to the consultant with the peptic ulcer.

(3) *Therapeutic diets* — an essential part of treatment not confined to the acutely ill in general hospitals.

(4) *Religion and culture* — beliefs and obligations often have nutritional significance and are certainly powerful influences. It is important that reasonable provision is made for minority groups.

It is important to bear in mind that about 18% of all patients are in the geriatric category and also that many elderly people are cared for by other specialists. Often poor appetite and severe discomfort lead them to take very small quantities. For such people at least something of what they like is better than meals that might be judged 'good for them' and remain uneaten. The impact of general nutrition concepts was made, on them, some years ago and now it is their special needs that must receive careful attention. A choice of dishes similar to that for younger people should be available so that soft or minced food need only be taken when necessary.

Of the remaining patients more than half are receiving psychiatric care. As the large institutions are reduced in size and people are accommodated in smaller units, greater effort will be needed to ensure that food and nutrition receive due priority. Thus, less than 40% of patients are in the medical, surgical and maternity categories and some 10% of those are likely to be prescribed modified diets. Modified diets are of course subject to change in the light of current nutrition and health concepts. In that acute sector the length of stay might be eight days or so. For perhaps four or five of those days, meals will be an important and emotive part of the total scene. In that time the hospital caterer can introduce or reinforce concepts of nutrition by the menu offered and, where appropriate, by including advice and explanation on the menu.

There are small categories of patients where application of the best nutritional advice is of greater importance or indeed essential, for example, for the younger disabled. People treated in metabolic units, renal units and so on have special needs.

There are people from a wide range of different trades and professions who contribute to the care of patients. The caterer depends on many of them and their managers. Most obviously, porters and drivers, nurses and ward domestic staff, less obvious perhaps, engineers, supply staff, treasurers and general administrators. In particular, nurses can help by assisting patients in their choice of food and by seeing that they receive it, that it is presented pleasantly and, when necessary, by helping the patient to eat. It would help to make further improvements if more doctors showed interest in their patients' food.

In many parts of the country, and nationally, action is being taken on the nutritional specification of food, especially factory prepared items. This has increased in importance as catering systems change and more prepared or 'manufactured' dishes are used in the menus. It is not always easy to specify. For example, in order to control the consumption of salt we have to consider not only salt added as such but also that in the ingredients of the formulation, both occurring naturally and used as a carrier for, say, flavours and seasonings. The significance of the whole and the parts has to be assessed and the methods of analysis or other checking have to be considered. The effect of substitutes for sodium is not being ignored and perhaps we should know more about the effect of chlorine.

The increase in consumption of wholemeal bread came more readily, although a few years ago it was difficult to obtain sufficiently competitive contracts. The bakery industry responded rapidly as public demand coincided with need of the hospital service. There are, of course, many people who prefer some white bread and can still have a diet conforming with current guidance.

The impact of present nutrition concepts is such that caterers and dietitians working in the DHSS have enlisted the help of colleagues within and outside the NHS in revising publications. For example, *Nutrition and Modified Diets* is in the final stages of revision. Work has started on *Health Service Catering — Standard Recipes* and it is envisaged that publication will be on cards suitable for the kitchen environment and in computerised form. The possibilities of 'view data' have not been overlooked. Volume 6, *Catering for Minority Groups*, will be re-examined and the assistance of anyone concerned with the nutritional needs of the Chinese communities in Britain would be welcomed.

The *Health Service Catering Bulletin*, now being printed, is mainly concerned with healthy eating. More specific guidance for hospital and welfare caterers is in prospect and it will be framed so as to be useful in the catering industry at large.

More locally, caterers in the Regions and Districts are in the throes of a competitive tendering exercise that invites tenders for catering by contract from commercial organisations for comparison with similar tenders generated 'in house'. The very first section of the model tender document draws attention to the *contract requirement* 'to meet the nutritional need of all patients' and to work in close liaison with the hospital dietitian over all catering. It also points to the need for the commercial tenderers to have the services of their own qualified dietitian. That guidance is also serving to remind caterers and dietitians already in post of the importance of this aspect of their day-to-day work.

A recent 'Rayner'-type scrutiny has resulted in all Authorities being told that they should institute catering performance reviews and a system developed in the Wessex Region is commended. That system includes nutritional standards expressed in terms of menu items. They embody the essence of recent reports and should be modified in the light of new knowledge as it becomes established. Performance reviews should be continuous. All Districts had to report to their Regions who were asked to summarise their reports and send them to the DHSS by December 1985.

An important impact on hospital catering has been to highlight training needs, sometimes to correct existing deficiencies (and these stretch across a wide spectrum of professions) and to provide updating. For catering staff and management the provision of suitable training is the responsibility of the recently established NHS Training Authority with various advisory groups. Meanwhile, the nutrition content in existing courses is being suitably amended without detracting from the core of conventional wisdom. An item of particular interest is our training package on *Nutrition* and *Modified Diets* that is in widespread use. It is intended mainly for in-service training of catering staff but can also be used with other disciplines. The sections start off with 'normal nutrition', including 'food composition' and 'a healthy diet'. It goes on to the 'needs of different groups', 'modification of texture', and, of course, an important content on 'modified diets'. The format is flexible enough to allow variations in presentation to meet local needs.

It is those local needs that matter and it is there that the results of the impact show in practical, hopefully constructive, ways. Menu planning, food specification and procurement, recipe selection, storage, preparation and cooking methods, distribution systems, equipment specifications and indeed novel 'total catering' systems are all receiving attention. Economic and political factors are powerful motivators but I hope that I have demonstrated that nutrition and health concepts do have an appropriate impact in responsible and responsive hospital organisations.

8
A 10-year study of nutrition and health in old age

R. SKINNER

ABSTRACT

Marked changes in the age structure of the population of the United Kingdom are taking place which are resulting in a significant increase in the number of elderly people, particularly the very old. These demographic changes have important implications for the provision of services for the elderly. For various reasons the elderly are considered to be a group at greater potential risk from under-nutrition than younger people, and the Department of Health has carried out several surveys of the elderly as part of its responsibility for nutritional surveillance.

In 1968 a nutritional survey of men and women aged 65 years or over was carried out in four areas of England and two areas in Scotland. Only subjects who were living in their own homes or with relatives were included and not those living in institutions.

Each subject was asked to keep a 7-day weighed dietary record, respond to a socio-economic questionnaire, have a medical examination and provide a sample of blood for biochemical and haematological analysis. 879 subjects took part, of whom 764 participated fully. Full details of the sample and analysis were published in 1972.

Five years later the survivors of the first survey were asked to take part in a repeat survey. A cross-sectional analysis of the 365 subjects who had responded fully in both surveys was published in 1979.

DISCUSSION

Although the theme of this book is catering, I am not writing specifically about catering for the elderly as I am not qualified to do so. Instead, I wish to discuss some of the findings from the various surveys of the elderly the Department of Health has carried out over the years, which I think have some relevance to the nutritional needs of the elderly and, therefore, catering. In particular, I shall be referring to information collected on subjects who had been surveyed on three separate occasions since 1967.

Marked changes in the age structure of the population of the United Kingdom are taking place which are resulting in a significant increase in the number of elderly people. The 1981 census showed that there were just over 7 million people aged 65 years or over in England. By the year 2011 the number is expected to increase to 7.7 million. Within this total considerable increases in the proportion of those aged 75 years or over are expected, as more and more elderly people live longer (Table 8.1).

These demographic changes have important implications for the provision of services for the elderly. It is therefore important that we learn more about the needs of the elderly. For various reasons the elderly are considered to be at greater risk of undernutrition than young people, the risk being greater with increasing age.

Table 8.1 Estimate of elderly population 1981–2011 (millions) by year and age group

Age	*1981*	*1991*	*2001*	*2011*
65+	7.108	7.463	7.339	7.609
75+	2.761	3.291	3.458	3.439
85+	0.511	0.730	0.897	1.003

In the 1960s, a programme of nutritional surveillance of at risk groups, including the elderly, was started by the Department of Health. A series of surveys of the elderly was started in 1967 with the following aims:

(1) to assess the nutritional status of elderly people living in private households;
(2) to investigate the relationship between nutrition and health in old age;
(3) to identify overt malnutrition and to determine factors which might be useful indicators of risk of malnutrition;
(4) when there is malnutrition, to identify related socio-economic factors in addition to dietary and medical factors;
(5) to elucidate the relative contributions of environmental factors, ageing and disease to malnutrition in the elderly;
(6) to study changes related to nutrition which occur with ageing and to find out how far these changes can be attributed to senescence and how far to disease processes;
(7) to contribute to our knowledge of how the physiological requirements for energy and nutrients change with age;
(8) to contribute to our knowledge in the elderly of reference ranges for biochemical and haematological investigations which are related to nutrition;
(9) to determine if there are any factors, besides age, which can be used in predicting mortality;
(10) to make recommendations in the light of survey findings.

The aims most relevant to this chapter are (3) and (7).

Longitudinal sample

In 1967–1968 a nutrition survey of men and women aged 65 years or over was carried out in six areas of Great Britain. The choice of areas was governed by practical considerations, including that there was a senior physician in geriatric medicine in each of the areas who was interested in the aims of the study and willing to co-operate.

The areas chosen were Cambridgeshire, Camden, Portsmouth and Sunderland in England and Angus and Rutherglen in Scotland.

A random sample of men and women who were aged 65 years or over was drawn from the registers maintained by the local Executive Councils for the administration of the National Health Service in each area, except Camden. The sample was weighted in favour of men and of the more elderly so that approximately equal numbers of men and women in each of the two age groups, 65–74 years and 75 years or over, were included. Both urban and rural areas were included, but the sample was not necessarily representative of Great Britain. In each area, only subjects who were living in their own homes or with relatives were included, and not those living in institutions.

Each subject was asked to keep a 7-day weighted dietary record, to respond to a socio-economic questionnaire, to have a medical examination and to provide a blood sample for biochemical and haematological analysis (Table 8.2). 879 subjects took part in the survey, of whom 764 participated fully. Full details of obtaining the sample and the response have been described and the results analysed (DHSS, 1972).

Table 8.2 DHSS surveys of the elderly 1967–68 to 1978

Areas	
England:	Cambridgeshire, Camden, Portsmouth, Sunderland
Scotland:	Angus, Rutherglen
Methods	
Dietary:	7-day weighed records
Medical:	Clinical examination
Radiological:	X-ray, left hand
Biochemical:	Total serum protein, serum albumin, pseudocholinesterase, Ca, P, alkaline phosphatase, leucocyte ascorbic acid, red cell transketolase
Haematological:	Haemoglobin, serum and red cell folate, serum B_6, serum B_{12}, serum Fe, total iron binding capacity
Socio-economic:	Questionnaire

Five years later, in 1972–1973, all but three of the participants in the first survey were traced; 277 had died. The survivors were asked to take part in a repeat survey. Some information was obtained from 483 subjects living in private households and full information from 379. 365 subjects responded fully in both the surveys and the 1972–1973 findings for these subjects have been analysed cross-sectionally (DHSS, 1979).

In 1977–1978 the subjects who took part in the 1972–1973 survey were again traced. Information was obtained from general practitioners, the local Family Practitioner Committees, Registrars of Deaths and the Office of Population Censuses and Surveys. The survivors who had participated fully in the two previous surveys, and who were still living in private households, were asked to take part in a third survey. The results of the tracing are shown in Table 8.3. Four subjects were traced but not contacted; one of them was known to have moved out of the area and the other three were in hospital or too ill to take part. 154 subjects participated fully, i.e., 20% of the 764 full participants in 1968.

Thus, the full range of information was obtained for each of these 154 subjects at each of the three surveys, i.e., in 1967–1968, 1972–1973 and 1977–1978. For convenience the survey is described as having taken place in 1968, 1973 and 1978.

Table 8.3 The origin of the 1978 sample from the subjects who participated fully in both the 1968 and the 1973 surveys

	Number of subjects (all areas)	
Full response in 1968 and 1973	365	
Died between 1973 and 1978	138	
Not traced in 1978	11	
Traced but not contacted	4	
No longer living in private household	9	
Eligible subjects asked to participate	203	(100%)
Full response	154	(76%)
Partial response	38	(19%)
Refusal	11	(5%)

As mentioned above, the sample was designed to give approximately equal numbers of men and women in each of the two age groups, age 65–74 years and age 75 years or over. As would be expected, subjects who were in the older age groups in 1968 were less likely than those in the younger age groups to have survived and taken part in the later surveys. For example, of the men who were aged 65–74 years in 1968 and who were full participants in that survey, 27% (56/205) took part fully in both 1973 and 1978, compared to only 8% (13/173) of the men aged 75 years or over. Also the proportion of women in the sample increased slightly from 51% (386/764) in 1968 to 55% (85/154) in 1978. In 1978 all subjects were aged 75 years or over and the mean age was 81 years for both men and women. The men ranged in age from 75 to 95 years and the women from 75 years to 91 years.

Cross-sectional and longitudinal surveys

One of the aims of the surveys was to investigate changes with age in subjects aged 65 years or older. This can be done by comparing subjects of different ages at one point in time using a cross-sectional survey. Another approach is a longitudinal study in which repeated measurements are made on a group of subjects at intervals over a period of time.

The 1968 survey was designed as cross-sectional and the results of the 1973 survey were also analysed cross-sectionally. The two reports found many differences between the two age groups studied and these differences were usually interpreted as changes with age. For example, the older subjects had, on average, a lower energy intake than younger subjects. The most likely explanation was that subjects changed their intake with age due to a higher incidence of disease, decreased physical activity or some other reason and some evidence was found for this. However, other explanations are possible.

Let us consider the subjects who took part in the 1968 survey and who were compared in two age groups, 65–74 years and 75 years or over. The two groups differed in that all the subjects in the older age group were at least 75 years old, but not all of the younger subjects were destined to reach this age. Some were to die between 1968 and 1978 before reaching the age of 75 years. One could postulate that energy intake was related to survival and that subjects who did not eat excessively were more likely to survive. Under this hypothesis, in a cross-sectional study, intakes of energy would appear to be lower in the older age group than the younger age group, even though the individual subjects did not change their intakes with age.

One could further propose that subjects born at different times may have grown up with different eating habits and these patterns may have been maintained throughout life. Subjects aged 65-74 years in 1968 were born in 1894–1903 and subjects in the older age group were born before 1894. Any differences between these two cohorts due to factors operating early in life would appear as an age difference between the two groups in a cross-sectional survey. For example, there was some evidence in the 1973 survey that the older age group was shorter than the younger subjects, which may be partly a cohort effect. We know from a recent survey of the heights and weights of 10 000 adults in Great Britain that in general older people are shorter than younger people (Rosenbaum *et al.*, 1985). On the basis of height this would suggest that the older subjects had lower energy requirements than the younger subjects. In summary, cross-sectional results give no information as to how *individuals* change with age.

One purpose of the surveys was to determine changes related to ageing. It was intended that the results from the 154 people who were full responders in all three surveys would be considered together to examine changes within individuals with age.

Unfortunately, there may be problems in interpretation of a longitudinal survey also. Even if a variable is found to change within an individual, this change is not necessarily due to ageing *per se*, but may be due to social or economic changes over the period of the survey. For example, elderly people in general may have been less active physically in 1978 than ten years previously, in which case they would have lower energy requirements. In addition, one must not overlook the problem of measurement at different times. For example, the assay for a biochemical variable may exhibit drift over a period of time, which may give rise to an apparent but spurious difference. For this reason, it is important that repeat measurements should be carried out by the same laboratory, or, in more general terms, that the methodologies used on separate occasions should be the same.

Findings from the longitudinal survey

Table 8.4 gives results for the average daily intake of energy. Longitudinal changes, within individuals, showed a significant decrease of energy intake with age. Cross-sectional studies have shown that older people eat less and the longitudinal study confirms this. The most probable explanation is decreased requirement, relating to decreased energy expenditure and decreased metabolic rate resulting from a decline with age in lean body mass (Debry *et al.*, 1977).

Intakes of animal protein, fat, calcium, niacin, vitamin D and

Table 8.4 Energy intake at each survey by age at first survey, for men and women separately

Energy intake (year)	*Age at first survey* 65–69	70–74	75–79	80+	*All ages*
Men					
1968	2445	2374	2274	1800	2378
1973	2245	2191	2066	2070	2190
1978	2088	2008	1874	1760	2015
No. of subjects	29	27	12	1	69
Women					
1968	1708	1912	1780	1146	1789
1973	1688	1701	1678	1064	1683
1978	1624	1838	1488	1057	1644
No. of subjects	36	30	18	1	85

pyridoxine decreased significantly with age. There were no significant changes in intakes of riboflavin, vitamin C or added sugars. Riboflavin is derived largely from milk and fortified breakfast cereal and the implication is that consumption of these foods, regardless of other changes in the diet, remained fairly constant. Since thiamin requirements are related to carbohydrate consumption and since thiamin is a constituent of many foods with a high carbohydrate content, the lowered intake does not appear to be a matter of concern. The iron and vitamin A contents of the diets of women decreased over the years. There was a slight decrease in the consumption of meat and green vegetables, which may have accounted for this.

The quality of the diet is better illustrated by expressing intakes of nutrients per 1000 kcal. The only significant decreases were fat intakes in both men and women and vitamin D and protein intakes in women. All other significant changes were in an upward direction, indicating an increase in nutrient density. One would expect that those nutrients which are energy linked, because of their wide distribution throughout foods common in the UK diet, would show a decrease in absolute terms but remain relatively constant per 1000 kcal. It is reassuring to find that those nutrients which are relatively independent of energy intake, because of the limited number of foods containing them (vitamins A, C and D), also remain constant or increase (except vitamin D in women).

It appeared that energy reduction had been achieved largely by restriction of foods containing relatively few nutrients, such as fat, and that eating patterns and the quality of the diet remained largely unchanged.

Evidence of malnutrition

The term 'malnourished' may be defined as any distortion of the form or function of an individual that could be due to an excess or deficiency of total food energy or of one or more nutrients. In relation to the Department's elderly surveys, the terms 'malnutrition' and 'undernutrition' have been used synonymously.

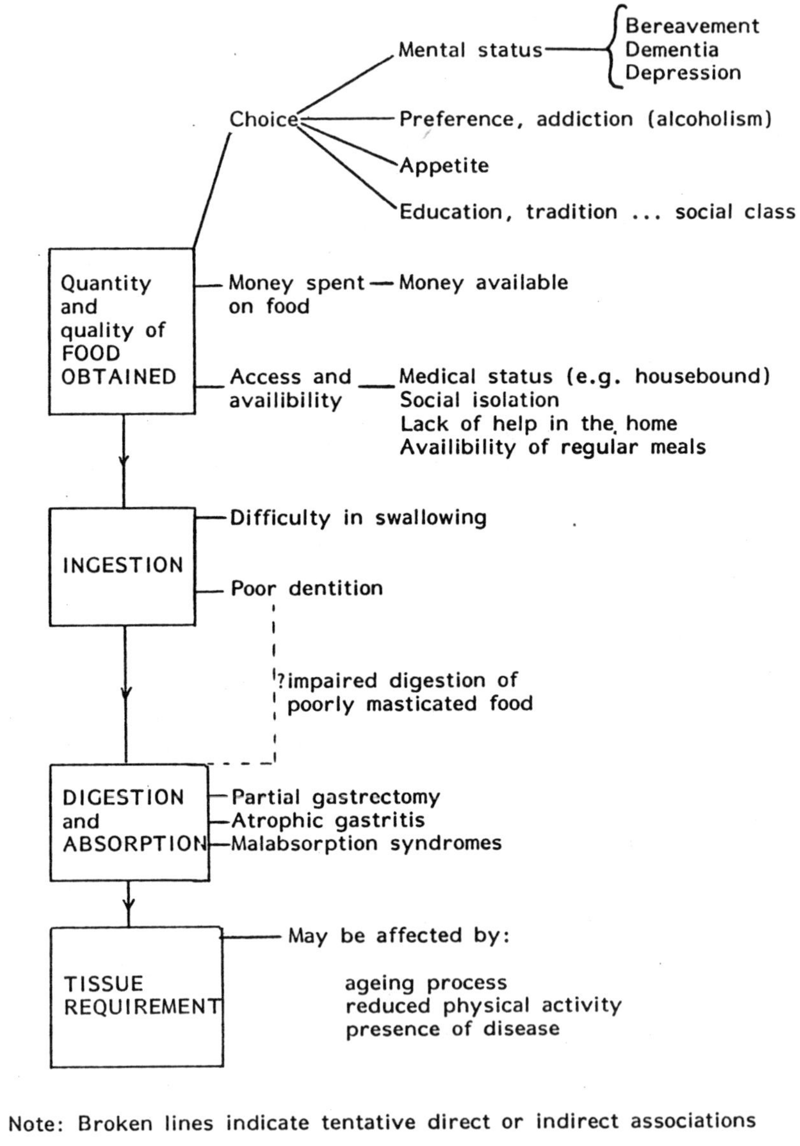

Figure 8.1 Inter-relationship of the factors which may influence the nutritional status of the elderly

Figure 8.1 outlines the inter-relationship of the various factors which may influence the nutritional status of the elderly. There are difficulties in making the diagnosis of malnutrition in the elderly due to the frequent co-existence of illness and to ignorance of the 'normal' changes occurring with age. Clinical signs are usually non-specific and laboratory results may be difficult to interpret.

The diagnosis of undernutrition was based on the clinical and dietary information and laboratory findings taken together, and, as far as possible, was consistent with the criteria adopted in the 1973 survey. Table 8.5 lists the main risk factors for malnutrition derived from the 1973 survey (DHSS, 1979).

Table 8.5 Risk factors for malnutrition

Environmental:	Living alone No regular cooked meals Supplementary benefit Social classes IV and V
Medical factors:	Low mental test score Depression Chronic bronchitis and emphysema Poor dentition Difficulty in swallowing Housebound

Malnutrition occurred in 6% of subjects (9/154) in 1978 compared with 7% (23/365) found in the 1973 survey, although a few included in 1978 were only marginally malnourished. Since disease processes are normally major factors contributing towards malnutrition, the incidence of malnutrition might be expected to be higher in those who had survived ten years. On the other hand, the 154 subjects who had taken part in all three surveys were, in some respects, a special group.

As in the 1973 survey, medical factors played an important role in seven out of the nine malnourished subjects in the 1978 survey, and environmental factors contributed in five out of the seven. The remaining two had adopted unusual diets and neither medical nor environmental factors were considered important.

An important aspect of these surveys is to identify, where possible, factors which are amenable to correction. For medical problems this is not always possible in medical terms. The chronic diseases of old age are, in general, inevitable in their progression. However, dilation of an oesophageal stricture, for example, can give rise to immediate improvement and advances in drug therapy will lead to a reduction in the number of partial gastrectomy operations being carried out and, therefore, a reduction in the number of those at risk of the long-term sequelae of undernutrition from such operations. In subjects with dementia, some form of support is needed to ensure that they are eating properly. Similarly, for subjects with a physical impairment, help is necessary so that they are not disabled by their impairment but are able to cope with the normal demands of living.

Two subjects were malnourished from eating unusual diets of their own devising. Such people are more difficult to identify and are unlikely to draw attention to themselves by seeking health advice directly from health professionals. One can only recommend a policy on increased awareness in those dealing with the elderly to the possibility that there may be some who have unusual ideas about diet and health.

CONCLUSIONS

Perhaps I should end by drawing attention to some facts which have a bearing on this question of malnutrition. The increase in numbers of elderly in the foreseeable future will be largely confined to those over 75 years of age. After 75 the likelihood of physical or mental disability increases sharply. Loss of mobility, failing sight or hearing, instability and incontinence are common problems. Dementia is estimated to affect 13% of those over 75 and 22% of those aged 80 or over. 41% of those over 75 live alone. All those various factors have been shown to be related to malnutrition in the elderly. For those with responsibility for looking after and providing health care to the elderly, there is needed a continuous awareness of how these various medical and environmental factors can interact in any individual elderly person.

In conclusion, reasonably healthy elderly people do seem to eat less as they grow older and their reduced intake is a reflection of their energy expenditure. Nevertheless, they seem to maintain and, in many respects, improve the nutritional quality of their diets. This underlines the need in catering for the elderly to ensure that meals provided for them are of a high nutrient density apart from the obviously desirable properties of palatability and acceptability.

References

Debry, G., Bleyer, R. and Martin, J. M. (1977). Nutrition of the elderly. *J. Hum. Nutr.*, **31**, 195–203

Department of Health and Social Security (1972). *A Nutrition Survey of the Elderly*. Report on Health and Social Subjects, No. 3. (HMSO, London)

Department of Health and Social Security (1979). *Nutrition and Health in Old Age*. Report on Health and Social Subjects, No. 16. (HMSO, London)

Rosenbaum, S., Skinner, R. K., Knight, I. B. and Garrow, J. S. (1985). A survey of heights and weights of adults in Great Britain, 1980. *Ann. Human Biol.*, **12** (2), 115–27

Index